beyond āsanas

beyond
āsanas

THE MYTHS AND LEGENDS BEHIND YOGIC POSTURES

PRAGYA BHATT

PHOTOGRAPHY BY
JOEL KOECHLIN

PENGUIN
ANANDA

An imprint of Penguin Random House

PENGUIN ANANDA

USA | Canada | UK | Ireland | Australia
New Zealand | India | South Africa | China | Singapore

Penguin Ananda is part of the Penguin Random House group of companies
whose addresses can be found at global.penguinrandomhouse.com

Published by Penguin Random House India Pvt. Ltd
4th Floor, Capital Tower 1, MG Road,
Gurugram 122 002, Haryana, India

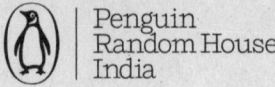

First published in Penguin Ananda by Penguin Random House India 2019

Text copyright © Pragya Bhatt 2019
Photographs copyright © Joel Koechlin 2019
Intext illustrations by Harryarts

ISBN 9780143446873

Typeset in Sabon by Manipal Digital Systems, Manipal

Printed at Manipal Technologies Limited, India

www.penguin.co.in

MIX
Paper | Supporting
responsible forestry
FSC® C043100

This is a legitimate digitally printed version of the book and therefore might not have certain extra finishing on the cover.

To all my teachers—
because of you, I'm a student
and
To all my students—
because of you, I'm a teacher

गुरुर्ब्रह्मा गुरुर्विष्णु गुरुर्देवो महेश्वरः
गुरु साक्षात परब्रह्मा तस्मै श्रीगुरवे नमः

Guru is the Creator, Guru is the Preserver, Guru is the Destroyer
Guru is the absolute Lord himself, salutations to that Guru

contents

foreword

Yoga. A form of exercise? Meditation for the spiritually advanced? A hippie trend? A way of life?

The word has been adopted and appropriated around the world many times over, and the practices tweaked and varied to suit different commercial or cultural settings.

Personally speaking, I have found my forms changing and evolving with time and experience in the practice, and believe that yoga is as much an inward journey as an outward achievement. This book offers lovely anecdotes from mythology, giving context to the names of postures, their reason for being, and includes step-by-step methodology for practicing each one and support them.

Is it not surprising that the meaning of asana names is seldom brought to light in yoga literature? In fact, these names have certainly not been chosen at random: whenever a name has been given to a specific asana, it has been designed to convey the essence of the asana, its spirit, so to speak. The physical description of an asana and the modus operandi to achieve the posture are, of course, important. But the physical part is only half of it. Yoga is not just some sort of exotic practice of gymnastics. If the combination of spirit, mind and psychological attitude is ignored, a large part of the asana's power is lost. *Beyond Asanas* superbly fills the gap with a beautiful visual story set to the backdrop of Hampi that conveys the character of an ancient wisdom.

Enjoy!

Kalki Koechlin

what is yoga?

MEANING AND ORIGIN

The term 'yoga' comes from the Sanskrit root *yuj*, which means to yoke together, to bind, to join or to attach. Yoga is a set of practices that result in the union of the individual self with the universal self. The earliest mention of yoga is in the Rig Veda, the first philosophical text of Hinduism.

Yoga has always been taught in the *guru-shishya parampara*, a system of learning where teachings are handed down from teacher to student and so on. Guru is a Sanskrit word. *Gu* means darkness. *Ru* means light. A guru is someone who guides a student (the *shishya*) from the darkness to the light. In ancient India, students lived with their gurus and learned yogic practices in the guru's ashram.

Yoga was practiced long before it was first documented. It was prevalent as a way of life. Because yoga was a largely oral tradition, it is difficult to date its origins. We can roughly date the origin of yoga to anywhere between 5000 and 10,000 years ago.

There is extensive Vedic literature about yoga. The three main texts on yoga philosophy are

- *Gheranda Samhita*
- *Shiva Samhita*
- *Hatha Yoga Pradipika*

Of these, the *Hatha Yoga Pradipika* is widely read by beginners and advanced students alike. It was written by Swamy Swatmarama in the fifteenth century. It contains comprehensive information on methods of body purification (*kriya*), pranayama, asana, *bandha* and mudra, among other topics. These comprise what we call 'Hatha' yoga. Hitherto, it was believed that 'hatha' was a combination of the word '*ha*', which means the sun, and '*tha*', which means the moon. However, recent research has shown that the word may simply mean 'force', referring to the vigorous style it is practised in. All modern styles of yoga can be clubbed under the umbrella of Hatha yoga.

PATANJALI'S *YOGA SUTRAS*

Another seminal yogic text is the *Yoga Sutras* of Patanjali. It is the most widely translated ancient Indian text in the world today. Patanjali was a sage who is believed to have lived in the second century BCE. The *Yoga Sutras* of Patanjali are a collection of 196 aphorisms about the practice and philosophy of yoga. The treatise is divided into four chapters:

- *Samadhi Pada*
- *Sadhana Pada*
- *Vibhuti Pada*
- *Kaivalya Pada*

According to the *Yoga Sutras*, the yogic path to enlightenment is an Ashtanga or Eight-Limbed path. The path consists of mental and physical challenges that ultimately lead the practitioner to moksha or enlightenment. The limbs of the Ashtanga system of yoga are:

- *Yama*—these are moral and ethical principles that must be followed by practitioners. The *yamas* include:

    - *Ahimsa*—non-violence. Yogis are expected to practise non-violence towards others and themselves.
    - *Satya*—truth. This goes beyond merely speaking the truth to having the courage to look beyond the perceived and convenient 'reality'.
    - *Asteya*—exercising control over one's desires and reducing one's wants. Yogis are expected to live austerely and focus on spiritual pursuits.
    - *Brahmacharya*—maintaining a disciplined sexual life. Contrary to popular perception, brahmacharya doesn't imply abstinence. Yogis are encouraged to practice discipline in sexual life, instead of uncontrolled indulgence.
    - *Aparigraha*—non-covetousness. Yogis should eschew excess and take only that which they need

- *Niyama*—these are rules that practitioners must live by to maintain purity in thought and deed.

    - *Saucha*—purity and cleanliness. Yogis are encouraged to maintain a clean body, a clean mind and clean surroundings.
    - *Santosa*—contentment. To practise being happy and satisfied rather than constantly looking at what is lacking teaches yogis equanimity.
    - *Tapas*—austerity. Yogis are encouraged to live simply and focus on their spiritual pursuits.
    - *Svadhyaya*—study of scriptures and of oneself.
    - *Isvara pranidhana*—surrendering to the supreme power.

- ◎ *Asana*—postures. The daily practice of yogic postures helps discipline the mind and the body.
- ◎ *Pranayama*—conscious inhalation, retention and exhalation of breath.
- ◎ *Pratyahara*—this is the practice of bringing the mind and senses under control by detaching oneself from the external world.
- ◎ *Dharana*—concentrating on a single point so that the mind remains calm and stable.
- ◎ *Dhyana*—dharana continued for a long time. In this phase, practitioners engage in self-study, reflection and keen observation of their physical and mental states. This is also the phase where body, mind, intelligence, will, consciousness, ego and self integrate.
- ◎ *Samadhi*—dhyana continued for a long time. When the practitioner reaches this phase, they are always peaceful.

Practitioners spend years studying and gaining perfection in each limb or stage of the Ashtanga path before progressing to the next one. In time, the seeker gains wisdom and ascends to samadhi.

adho mukha svanasana

(page 1)

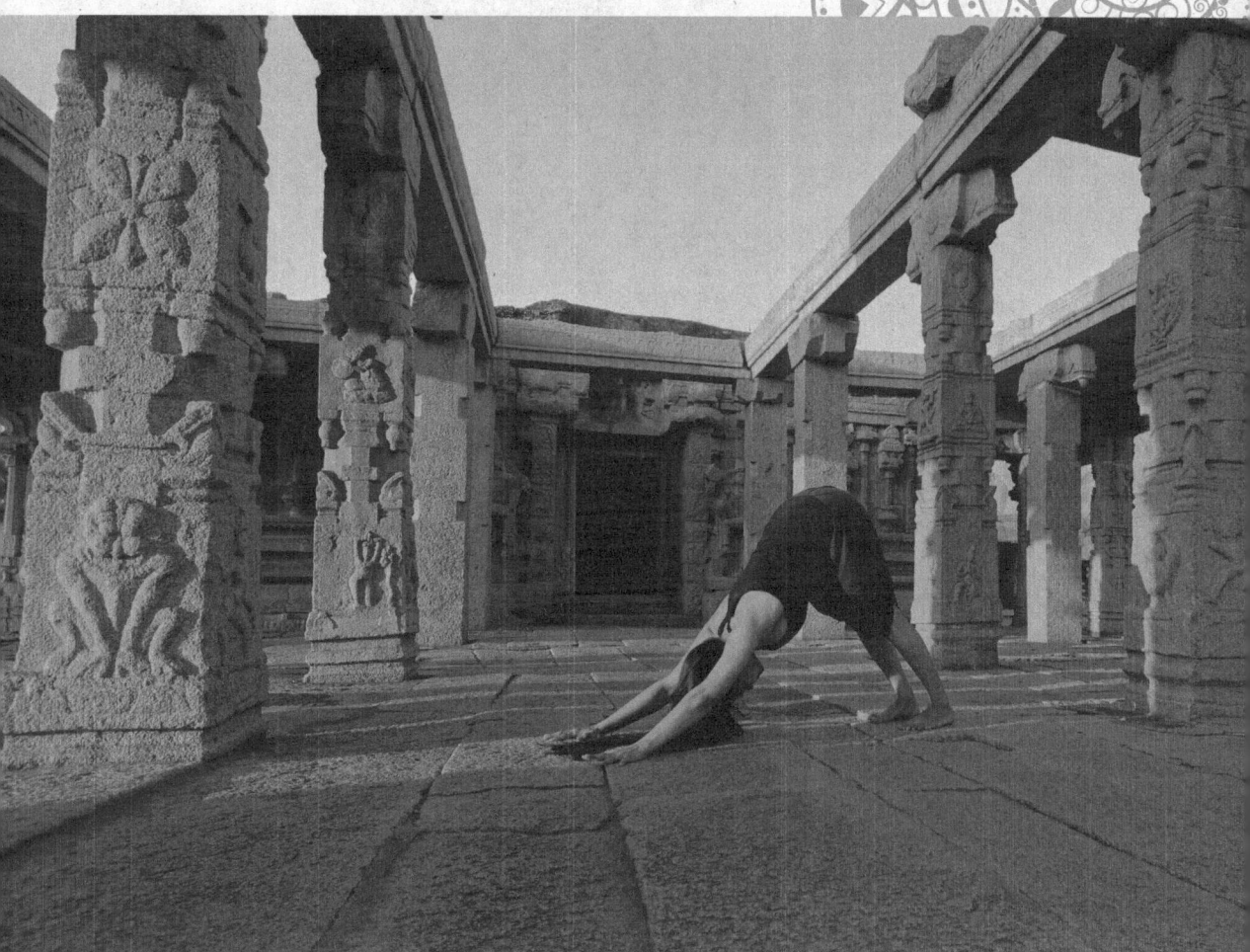

To be loyal and faithful in today's world, we need to be strong in our relationships and have the courage to forgive.

anjaneyasana
(page 7)

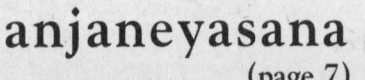

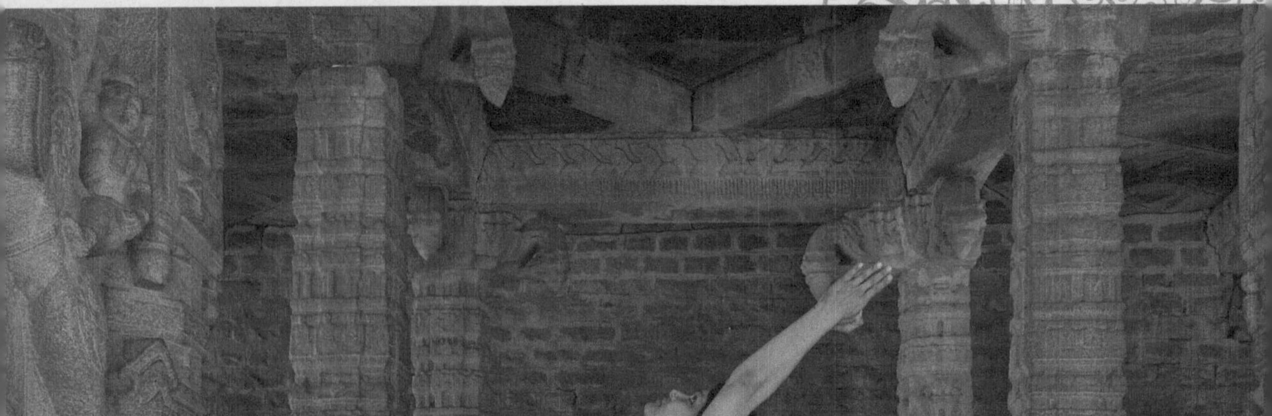

Our devotion to the practice, returning to the practice daily and belief in the system of yoga must be unwavering.

balasana
(page 12)

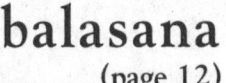

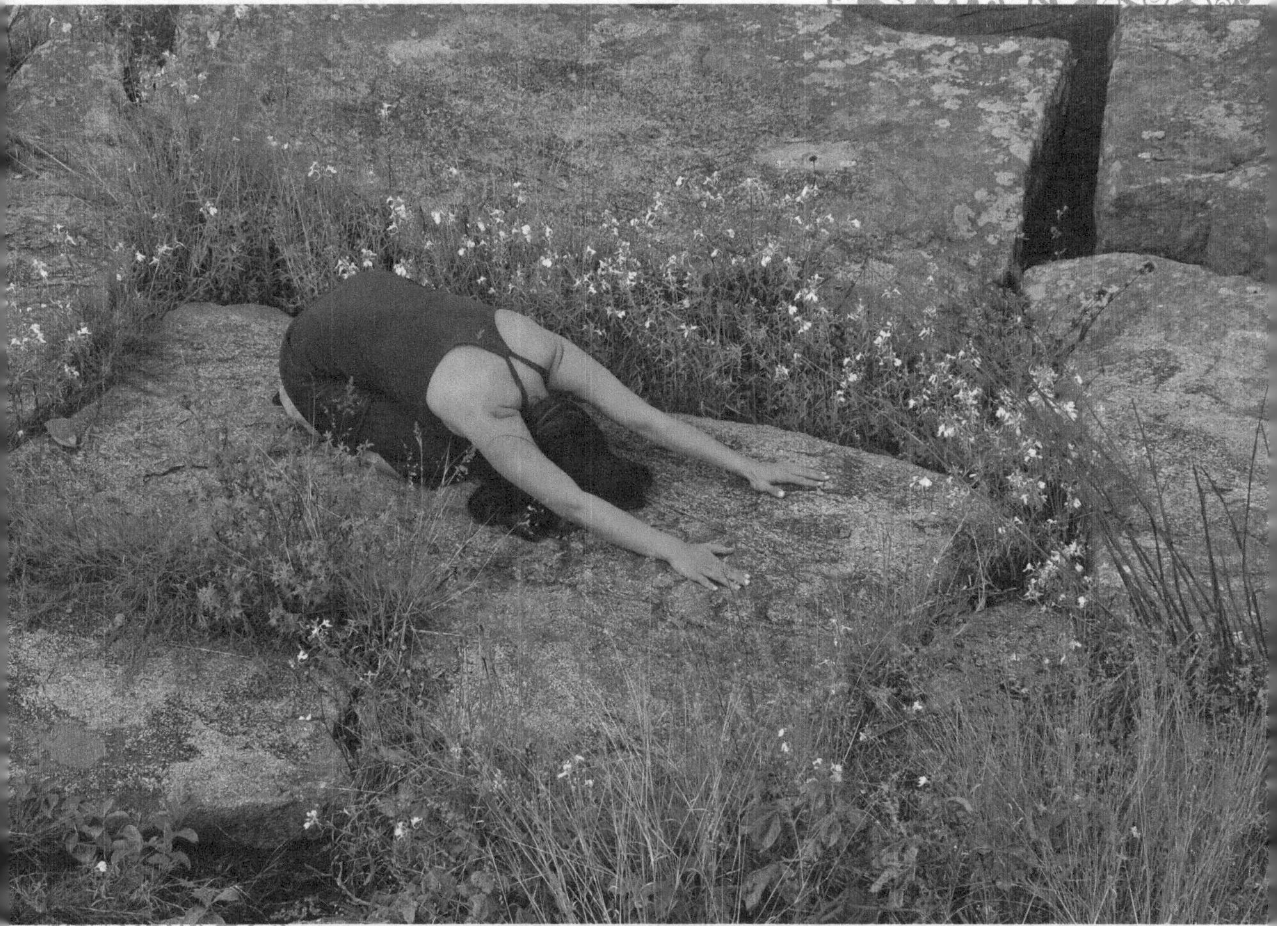

Everyone encounters roadblocks and setbacks, but those who move forward with courage get closer to their goals than those who lose hope. The path of yoga keeps us moving forward with vigour and strength.

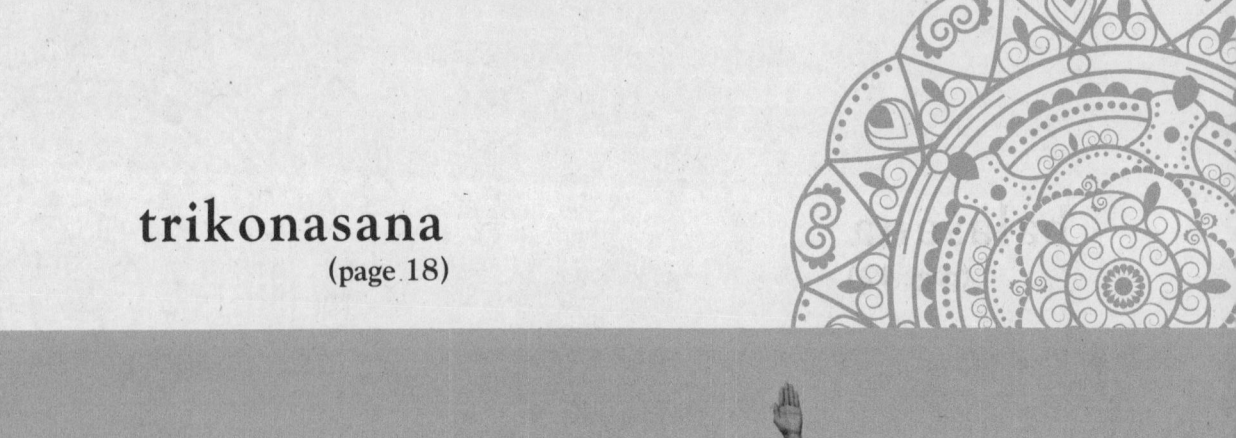

trikonasana
(page 18)

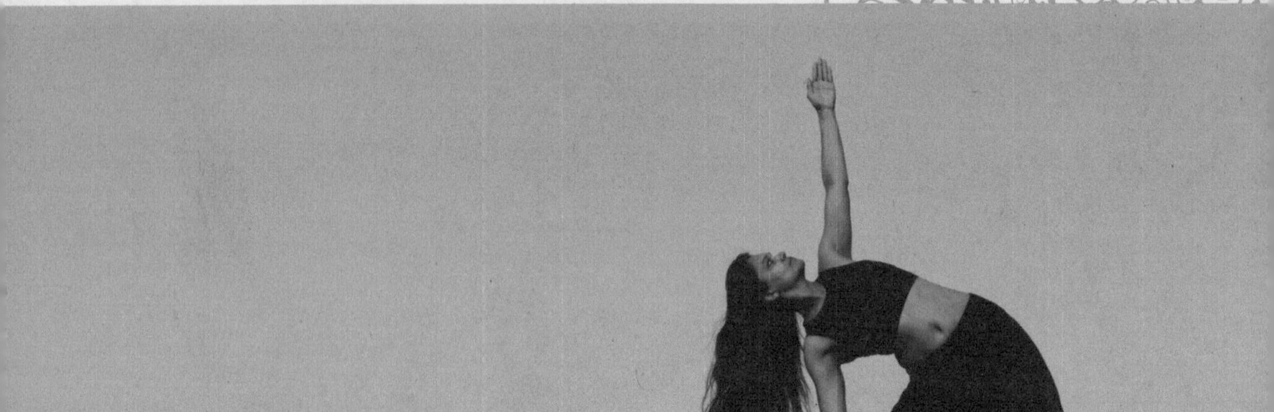

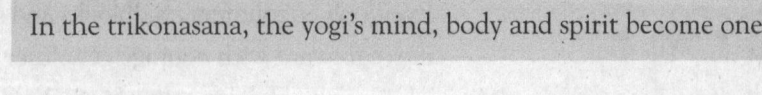

In the trikonasana, the yogi's mind, body and spirit become one.

ardha chandrasana
(page 24)

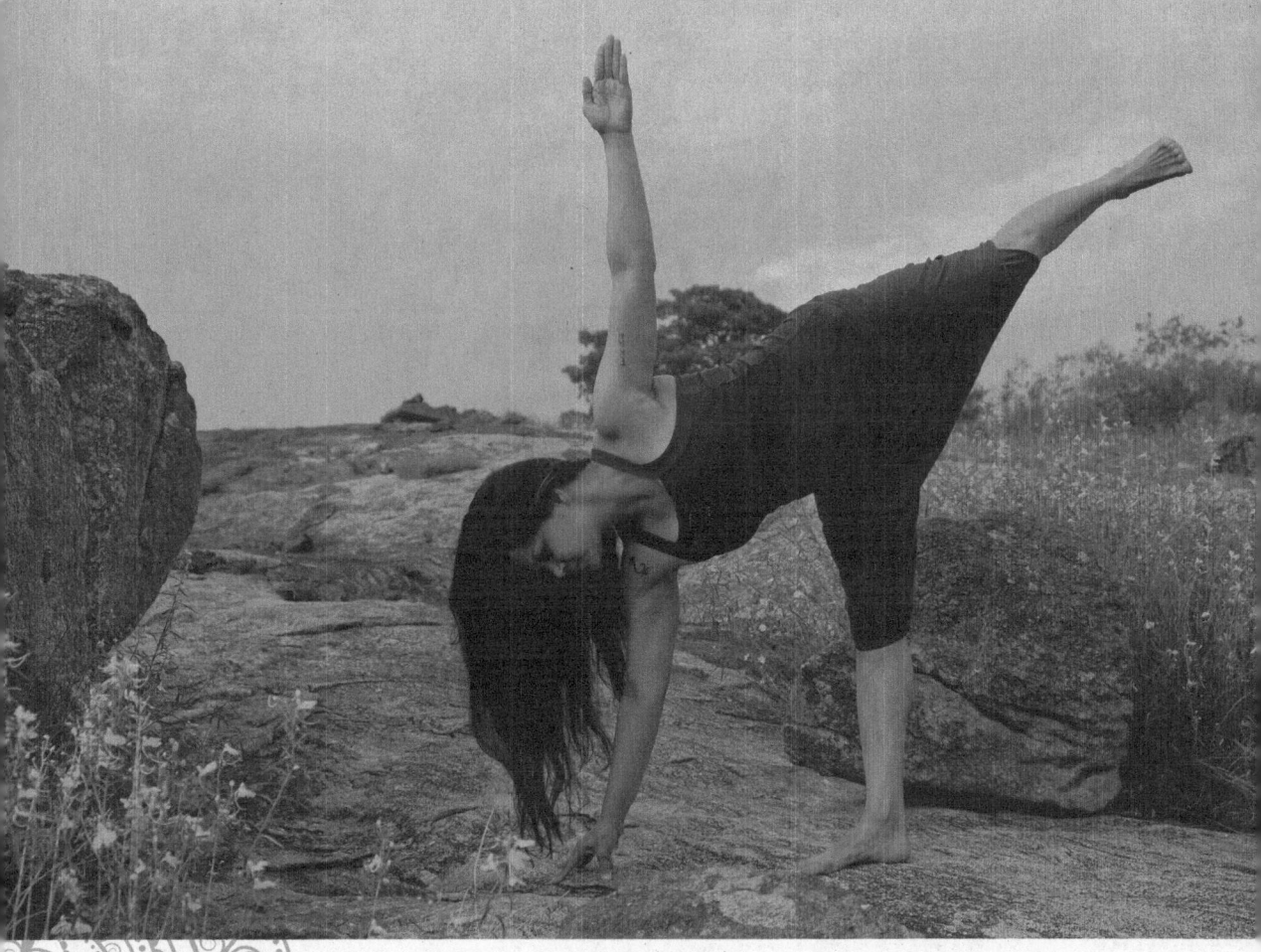

Rather than living in the past or in the perceived future, practitioners are encouraged to make peace with the present and to enjoy whatever it has to offer.

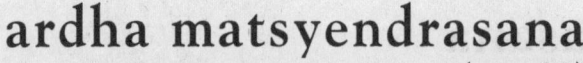

ardha matsyendrasana
(page 30)

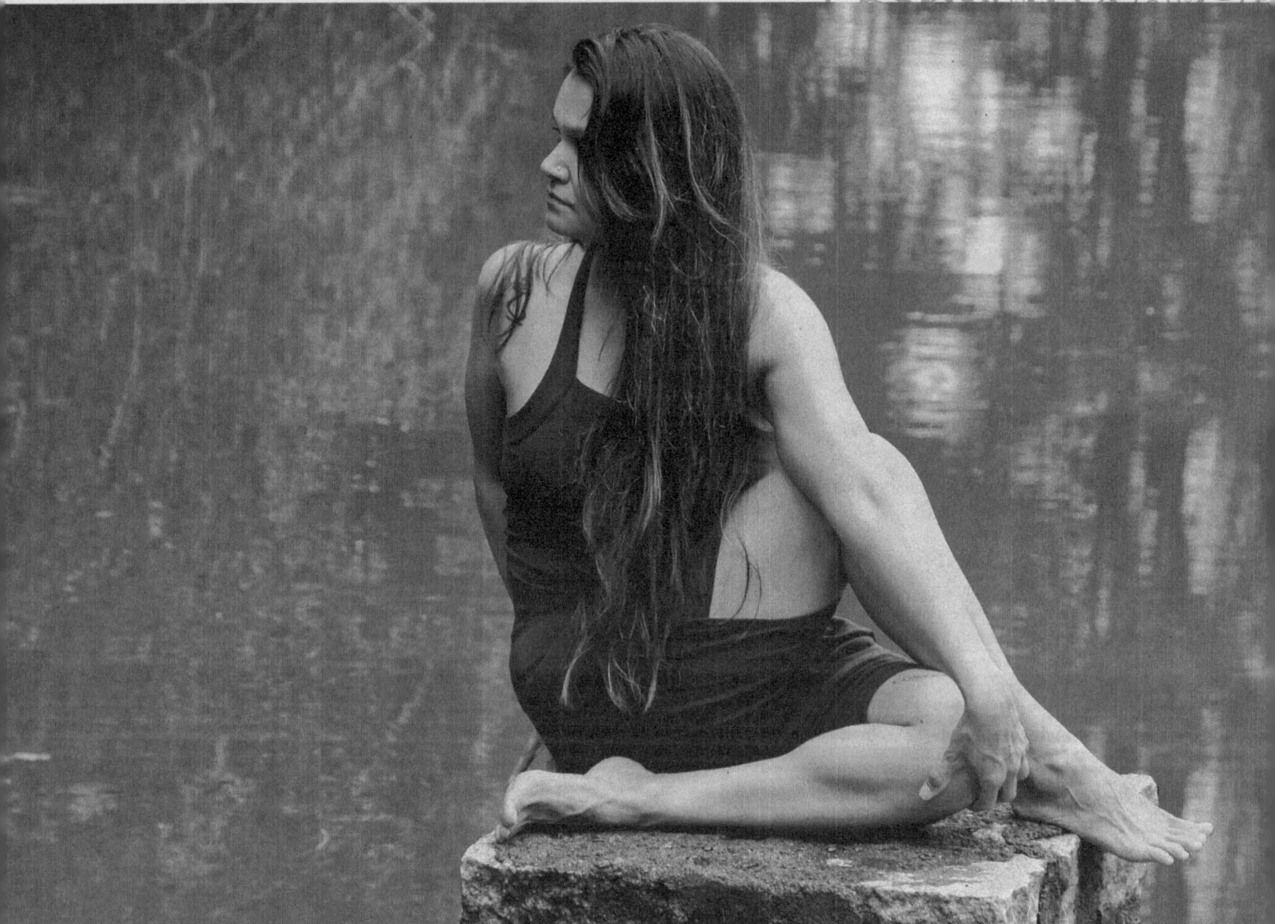

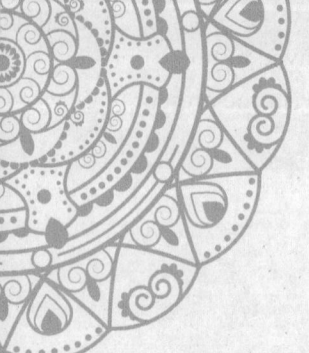

You will be able to look at your present and future without the fog of the past clouding your vision. You will experience clearer vision and perception.

kurmasana
(page 35)

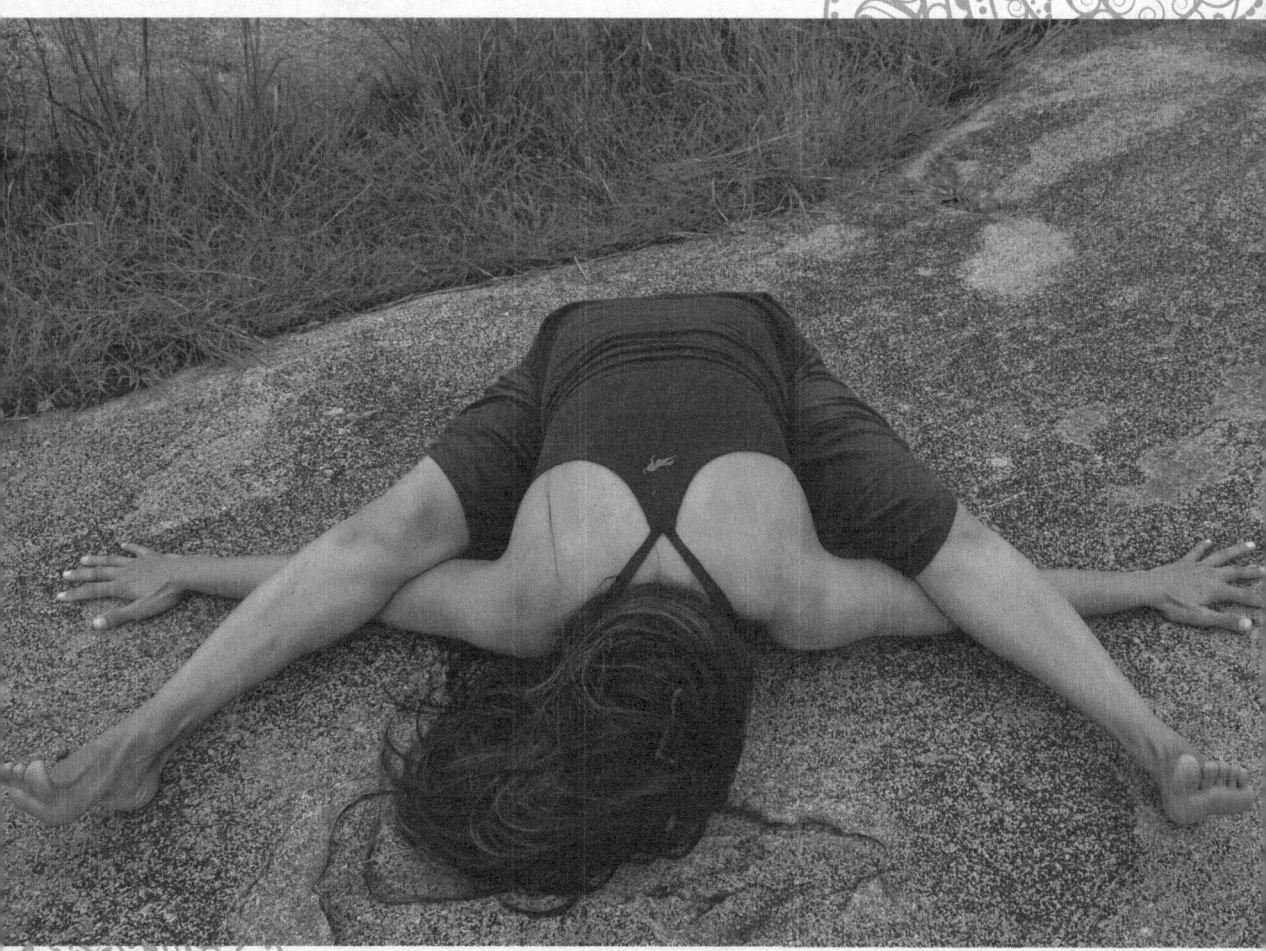

The tortoise withdraws into its shell to rest. Similarly, we need to recoup and rejuvenate at regular intervals to live life to our fullest potential.

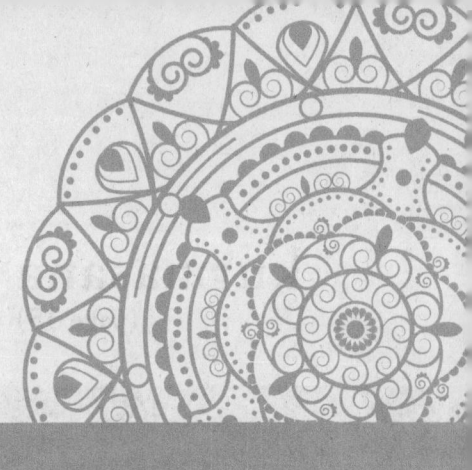

tadasana
(page 41)

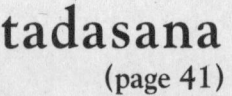

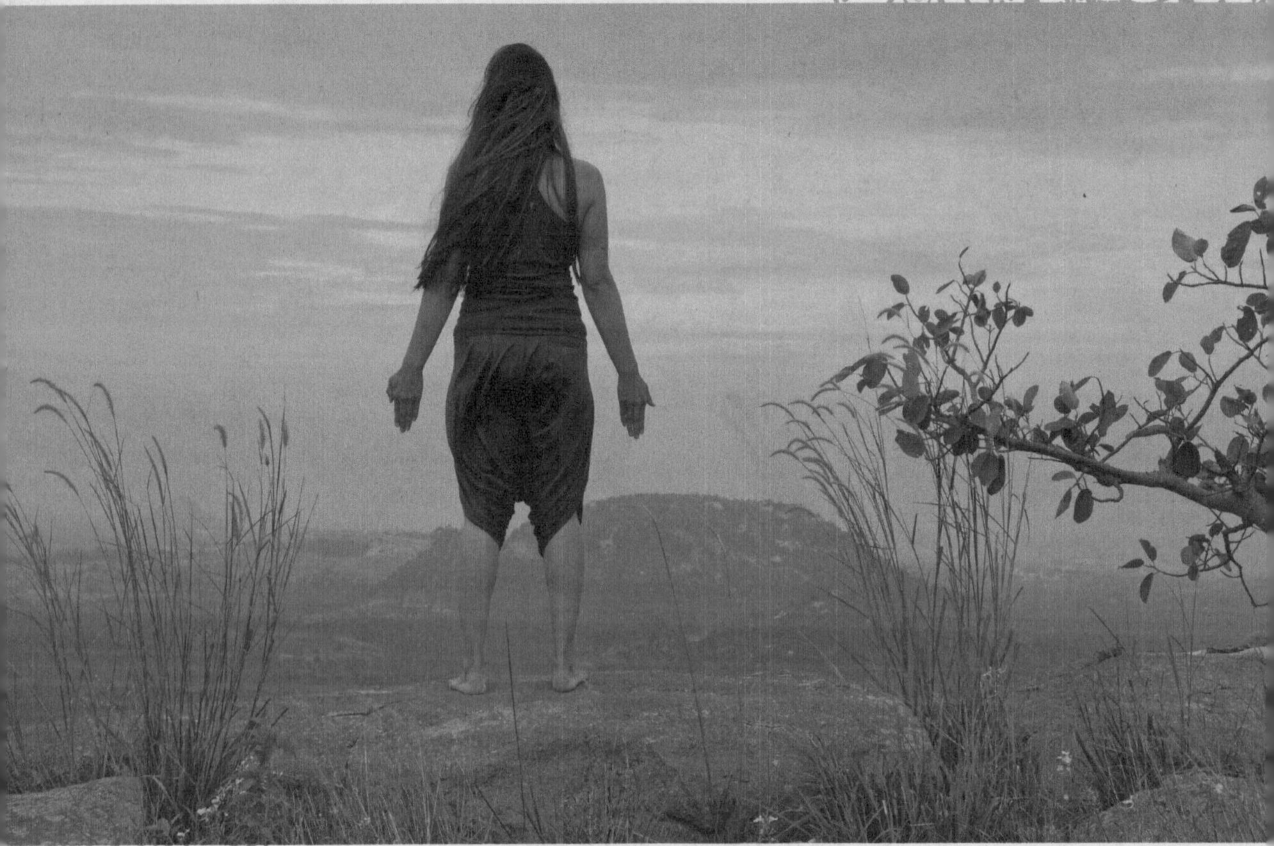

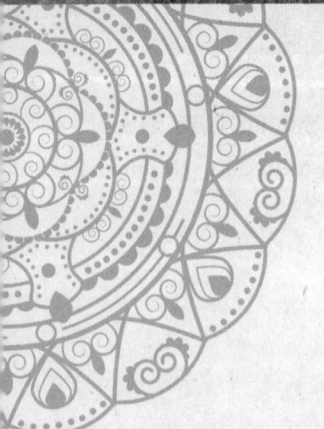

Before any movement, there has to be stillness, stability and balance. This pose calls for us to be steady and strong like a mountain.

1

adho mukha svanasana

(downward-facing dog pose)

The practice of yoga was neither 'invented' nor 'discovered'. It existed long before references to it first appeared in art and literature. Nature played an important role in rites and rituals, with ancient yogis drawing inspiration from the world around them. Almost all mythological figures were associated with at least one animal. It is no surprise, then, that many yoga poses are inspired by animals, insects and nature.

One such pose is the *adho mukha svanasana*. A careful study of the name tells us its meaning. '*Adho*' = Down; '*Mukha*' = Face; '*Svana*' = Dog; '*Asana*' = Pose.

FINDING THE HOLY COWS

Lord Indra was proud of being a capable and just leader. He ruled his kingdom, Indralok, fairly and never denied help to anyone. Lord Indra resolved all problems and disagreements promptly by holding court regularly. His subjects felt safe and secure. Anyone could present their problems to him and seek justice while the court was in session.

One story of such a day in court goes like this: One day, a group of cowherds came into Lord Indra's court. They complained that all their cattle had been stolen by some fearsome demons. Despite searching day and night, they found no trace of the cattle. They implored Lord Indra to help as their livelihood had been snatched away. 'You shall have your cattle back in no time,' Lord Indra assured them.

He promptly sent a few soldiers out to search for the cattle. After some time, they came back empty-handed, with no news.

Next, he sent even more skilled and formidable soldiers. They were adept at tracing lost things and people even in the densest jungles. After some time, they too came back empty-handed.

Then, Indra decided to send Suparna to survey the land aerially. Suparna was a supernatural bird and perhaps, from her vantage point, she would find some clue about the cattle's whereabouts. However, Suparna also came back with no information.

Now Indra was puzzled and the cowherds had started to despair.

Finally, Indra decided to call on Sarama for help. Sarama was a dog Indra relied on heavily whenever in need. She was swift-footed and had a strong sense of smell, which helped her find anything easily.

She sniffed around the area the cows had been grazing on. She made her way around the cowherds' settlement and sniffed there too. When she was unable to detect anything, she moved on to the rest of the jungle. She kept her sense of hearing and smell alert. However, she still couldn't find anything. Sarama continued going deeper into the jungle until she finally began to sense something. She quickly followed the trail and discovered the cows hidden in a remote cave. All this searching had made her hungry and to her delight, she also found food in the cave.

She quickly ran back to Lord Indra's court and guided him back to the cave. Everyone was overjoyed.

Sarama's happiness knew no bounds. She was glad to have served Lord Indra again and been of use to those who needed help.

A CONSTANT COMPANION

When the war of Kurukshetra in the Mahabharata was over, the Pandavas made their way to heaven. Slowly and quietly they ascended the mountain from where they would board the chariot to heaven. The eldest Pandava, Yudhishthira, led the way. He was followed by Bheema, Arjuna, Nakula, Sahadeva and Draupadi. A lone dog also followed them.

The journey up the mountain was long and arduous. They were all very tired. Soon, Draupadi collapsed and was unable to continue. The Pandavas looked at her with sorrow since she would not enter the kingdom of heaven. Throughout her life, Draupadi had secretly favoured Arjuna. This attachment to him had been her undoing.

The remaining Pandavas continued, even though their exhaustion increased with every step. The dog followed.

The next to collapse was Sahadeva. He had been proud of his own intellect and this vice kept him from the kingdom of heaven. The remaining Pandavas trudged on as the dog followed, wagging its tail.

Nakula collapsed next. 'He was proud of his looks and wouldn't stop admiring himself,' explained Yudhishthira to the others. 'That's why he will also not make it to the kingdom of heaven. Let us continue.' Yudhishthira had noticed the dog and had started to consider it a part of their entourage.

Arjuna collapsed next. He would also not make it to heaven. His failing was that he was overconfident and conceited.

The summit of the mountain was close and though they mourned their siblings and wife, Bheema and Yudhishthira continued. The dog wagged its tail and followed them.

Finally, Bheema also collapsed. He was proud of his physical strength and ate too much, thought Yudhishthira. By now, he was almost delirious with hunger and thirst, but carried on. He was aware that it was only him and the dog now.

At the top of the mountain, Lord Indra descended with his chariot and invited Yudhishthira in to be flown to heaven. Yudhishthira was happy that the harrowing journey was finally coming to an end. But being righteous and just, he had one final request. 'Lord Indra,' Yudhishthira said, 'I can only come to heaven if this dog comes with me. He has followed us from the base of the mountain, and has been with me as

I lost every single one of my siblings and my beloved wife. He has been with me in sorrow, in happiness, in sadness and in bliss. He has seen me tired and hungry. Now, when I'm at the brink of heaven, I do not wish to abandon him.'

Lord Indra, of course, could not allow a dog into heaven, as dogs were considered inauspicious.

Yudhishthira found himself becoming increasingly emotional. 'Lord Indra, the dog has done nothing to harm anyone or anything. It has shown only the utmost loyalty, faith and love. I'm afraid if he can't enter heaven, then neither can I.' So saying, he turned away from the celestial chariot and started to walk away.

Lord Indra stopped Yudhishthira. 'Congratulations, Yudhishthira, you have passed the ultimate test,' he said. 'This dog is none other than Dharma, and you have shown that you have an intimate bond with Dharma. Welcome to heaven.'

As Yudhishthira boarded the chariot and flew to heaven, the dog turned into the God of Dharma.

SIGNIFICANCE AND SYMBOLISM

There are many more references to dogs in Hindu mythology. For instance, Bhairava, an avatar of Shiva, rides a dog. In fact, Bhairava not only rides dogs, but also keeps company with them.

Early yogis considered all life equal. If there are poses named after sages, then there are poses inspired by animals as well. Yogis observed a dog languidly extending the spine while keeping the rest of the body alert. They were curious about the benefits that humans could derive from this movement, and decided to mimic the natural movements of a dog.

A yoga pose is more than just a physical posture, and it is worthwhile to study its other aspects. While performing the adho mukha svanasana, we should think about the qualities that make the dog man's best friend. In both the myths above, we see that a dog's sense of loyalty and devotion makes it a valuable companion. It's a fact that people with pet dogs are happier and feel less lonely. Guard dogs evoke a feeling of security in their owners. In recent years, dogs have also been trained to help the physically and mentally challenged manage their daily lives.

Today, we tame and domesticate animals to control and use them for our purposes. Rarely do we sit and think about what we can learn from our pets and other animals.

While practicing the downward dog pose, meditate upon the strength and courage of a dog. To be loyal and faithful in today's world, we need to be strong in our relationships and have the courage to forgive. The decisions we make, and the manner in which we conduct our lives, should be reflective of this.

HOW TO

1. Place your hands and knees on the floor, shoulder and hip width apart.
2. Spread your fingers wide on the mat and press the hands down firmly.
3. Start to straighten your legs.
4. Lift and extend your tailbone up and out.
5. Extend the torso by extending the spine.
6. Lengthen the back of the legs as you push the heels into the floor.
7. Relax the neck, face and shoulders.

HELPFUL HINTS

- For help in extending the spine, rest your heels against a wall and push into the wall with the heels.
- By bringing your chest closer to the knees, the shoulders and back will become more straight.

BENEFITS

- Engenders a sense of calmness.
- The increased blood flow to the brain helps relieve depression and anxiety.
- Stretches the shoulder blades and joints.
- Strengthens the ankles and tones the legs.
- Alleviates heavy menstrual flow.
- Helps relieve digestive problems such as constipation and indigestion.
- Reduces lower back ache.
- Increases flexibility of hips, knees and ankles.
- Counters the effects of wear and tear caused by jogging, walking and other sports.
- Strengthens the arches of the feet and helps to treat flat foot.

CONTRAINDICATIONS

Asanas in which the blood flows towards the head instead of towards the feet are called 'inversions'. Since the adho mukha svanasana is an inversion it is advisable to exercise caution if you have high blood pressure or get frequent headaches. The flow of blood to the head can exacerbate the condition. For the same reason, don't practice this asana if you have a migraine. Be careful with this asana during pregnancy. Avoid it if you are feeling a little under the weather, giddy or nauseous.

2

anjaneyasana

(low lunge pose)

In Hindu mythology, Hanuman is the son of Anjana. Anjana was an apsara, a celestial nymph. He is so significant in Hindu mythology that there are several asanas dedicated to him. Translated literally, *anjaneyasana* means the asana of the son of Anjana.

THE FRUITS OF *TAPAS*

Anjana came to earth and married Kesari, the chief of the Vanar Sena or army of monkeys. Even after many years, however, they were unable to have children. As the years went on, Anjana and Kesari's desire for a child intensified. Since they wanted a child more than anything else, Anjana decided to do vigorous penance to appease the gods. She sat in prayer for many hours every day, with her palms open to receive a boon from the gods.

Finally, Lord Shiva noticed her tireless devotion and undying faith.

He blessed a few seeds and called upon Vayu, the God of Wind. 'I have blessed these seeds, Vayu. Please drift across Anjana when she is deep in prayer with her palms open, and drop these seeds in her palms.'

Vayu did as he was told.

Anjana was startled out of her meditation when she felt the seeds fall into her hands. She instinctively understood this was the answer to her prayers, and swallowed the seeds. To her delight, she soon bore Hanuman.

Hanuman was a precocious child, much to his parents' annoyance. He got into trouble frequently. He had been blessed by Shiva and delivered by Vayu, and therefore he was a demi-god and very powerful. But he was unable to understand the extent of his own power. His naughtiness sometimes disrupted the lives of humans on earth.

Anjana tried her best, but she was unable to maintain the necessary control over her child. Finally, she called a meeting of the elders in the community to discuss what they could do about Hanuman. After much deliberation, it was decided that Hanuman would live with Sugriva (the King of the Vanar Sena). Participating in the vigorous training routine of the army would teach him discipline and control.

Anjana was dumbstruck. 'There must be some other way,' she implored the elders. 'We have done so much tapas, penance, for a child and I won't be able to bear having him taken from me!'

The elders remained firm. They reasoned with her and recounted the mischief that Hanuman invariably got into. They made her realize that his pranks were affecting the entire world. 'Spending time in the army, with all the rigours of army life, will do him good,' they assured her.

Although Hanuman was a naughty boy, he was also a dutiful son. He was a little nervous and didn't relish the thought of living with a completely new family. But he finally decided that it might be fun and agreed to go.

Tearfully and with her heart breaking, Anjana had to finally give in.

Over the years, she found solace in the fact that her son accomplished great feats of valour, strength and courage. He was one of the bravest members of the Vanar Sena and its greatest warrior. Anjana's pain eventually faded and was replaced by pride in her son's accomplishments.

SIGNIFICANCE AND SYMBOLISM

Anjana had conceived a child after long years of arduous penance. To have to give him up must have been a nightmare. She was probably surprised by her own courage when she agreed to the decision of the elders and let her offspring go. But she found the requisite strength somewhere in the depths of her being. She put her own beliefs and emotions aside for the greater common good.

Hanuman also, at such a tender age, had to deal with leaving a loving family to live with strict disciplinarians. Such events can scar a child, but Hanuman retained his childlike curiosity, did the best he could, and triumphed. Both Hanuman and Anjana displayed courage in the face of sacrifice.

When practising this asana, we must search and connect to the faith that resides in the core of our being. As our tight muscles loosen up and we are able to delve deeper into this pose, our faith in ourselves also deepens.

Psychosomatically, we store our fears and insecurities in our hips. The hips house deep-rooted fears. Over time, these emotions become psychologically and physically restrictive. They manifest as tight hips. Tight and inflexible hip muscles lead to back pain, slipped disc, etc. When we practise the anjaneyasana, we are reaching into a space that is inaccessible in other asanas. Because it is such a deep stretch, it is painful and uncomfortable at first. But if you focus on breathing deeply, you will be able to persevere through the pain and attain an exquisite sense of relief.

Similarly, before we let go of a painful memory, it is important to come face to face with it.

The faith and devotion that Anjana displayed are reflective of a true yogini. Our devotion to the practice, returning to the practice daily and belief in the system of yoga must be unwavering.

HOW TO

1. Start with the adho mukha svanasana (see Chapter 1).
2. Step forward and place your right foot between your hands.
3. Place your hands on your waist and lift the torso so that the spine is perpendicular to the floor.
4. Continue to open the chest by drawing the shoulder blades together and drawing them closer to the ribcage.
5. Raise your arms and align the upper arms with your ears.
6. Explore your limits through deep inhalations, sinking further into your pelvis. Repeat with the left leg.

HELPFUL HINT

◉ It helps to place a bolster under the front foot. The added height enables you to stretch the groin, hips and legs further.

BENEFITS

◉ Stretches the hip joint and psoas muscles.
◉ Stabilizes the hips and the core. Expands the chest and enables better breathing.
◉ Increases shoulder flexibility.
◉ Releases deep-seated fears, trauma and insecurities, enabling the practitioner to emerge from the shadows of the past.

CONTRAINDICATIONS

This asana is an intense stretch for the lower body and requires extensive engagement of the legs. Therefore, if you are recovering from an injury to the knee, hip or ankle, it's best to avoid it until you are completely healed.

3

balasana

(child's pose)

Children were often revered as harbingers of good luck in ancient India. Even today, they are believed to be a form of divinity.

There is much to learn from children. Long ago in India, children were expected to fulfil their destinies and grow into the role awaiting them. Princes who would become kings were trained to be benevolent and fair right from childhood. They had great teachers for warfare, statesmanship, ethics and morality. These teachers left an indelible impression on the child. Long associations with the royal family gave teachers a chance to observe the children and guide them appropriately.

NO ORDINARY CHILD

Sometimes, it was obvious that a child was unique and meant for greatness in the future. Lord Krishna was one such child. His birth was fraught with danger.

Through divine intervention and the determination of his mother and uncle, he survived.

However, as Lord Krishna grew up, he became very naughty. His distressed mother was always trying in vain to discipline him. She constantly worried about him because his antics could get him into grave danger.

One day, when Krishna was a mere toddler, he was playing with his brother in the forest. The forest was lush with trees and fruits. The other children, including his brother, were able to reach up to pick the fruits from the trees and eat them, but Krishna was too small. All the children were very excited and in a playful mood, and no one heard Krishna asking for fruit. Krishna did the next best thing, which, to him, meant picking up some mud and eating it.

'No!' Balrama, his brother, screamed as he saw Krishna push fistfuls of mud into his mouth. But it was too late. Krishna was in big trouble. All the other children had run to their mother, Yashoda, to tell her what Krishna had done.

When Balrama and Krishna got home, they found a very angry Yashoda waiting for him.

'Krishna, your friends told me you ate mud while you were playing. Is that true?' she asked him.

Krishna stoutly denied this.

'Are you sure?' persisted Yashoda.

Krishna firmly nodded his head.

'Then open your mouth and let me see,' said Yashoda.

Krishna did as he was told and Yashoda gasped in disbelief. She didn't see any mud. She didn't even see a tongue or any teeth. She saw the entire universe in his mouth. She saw all the planets, the constellations and the stars. Yashoda stood transfixed as she realized that her child was no ordinary child. He had the strength and wisdom of the universe in him.

AN HONOURABLE STUDENT

In ancient India, class and caste divisions were enforced strictly. Eklavya was the son of a poor hunter in the forest.

The forest was in a crisis as the deer were being hunted by the leopards. The hunters were helpless because they didn't have the skills to hunt and kill leopards. The crisis was a great one, and Eklavya took it upon himself to find a solution.

He had heard of Dronacharya, the greatest archery teacher of all time. Eklavya went to Dronacharya and appealed to be taken on as a student. Eklavya didn't know it at the time, but Dronacharya was bound by the rules of the kingdom. Teachers of the royal family were not allowed to teach commoners. It was believed that there could be no warriors better than the kings and the princes of the kingdom. This ensured that if a violent uprising occurred, the princes could easily enforce peace and keep the kingdom safe.

'I'm sorry, Eklavya,' said Dronacharya. 'As much as I would like to teach someone as deserving as you, I am bound by the rules.'

Eklavya accepted this decision, although he felt it was unfair. But he was not disheartened. He decided to learn archery by only observing Dronacharya teaching. He made a clay statue of Dronacharya and placed it on a pedestal. He worshipped it daily like one worships a guru. He observed Dronacharya teaching the royal princes and practised those lessons himself. Through sheer hard work, dedication and perseverance, he became so adept that he could shoot an arrow with his eyes closed and not miss the mark!

One day, Arjuna and his brothers were hunting in the forest. Their dog was running ahead of them and barking very loudly. Suddenly, the dog stopped barking. The brothers were worried and rushed ahead to check on their dog. When they found him, they saw that his mouth was clamped shut with a number of arrows around the snout. The dog was unhurt, but was unable to bark. The brothers wondered if Dronacharya was nearby, since only he could shoot arrows with such precision.

They looked for Drona and instead, found Eklavya in the forest. Although he didn't really believe the answer would be yes, Arjuna asked Eklavya if he was responsible for clamping the mouth of the dog shut. To everyone's surprise, Eklavya said yes.

'Who taught you such amazing skills in archery?' asked Arjuna, confounded. 'These are skills far above and beyond those possessed by us in the royal family.'

'Drona taught me,' Eklavya said simply.

Arjuna's anger knew no bounds. He raced home and confronted Dronacharya. Dronacharya was, of course, utterly confused. He stated repeatedly that he had imparted training only to the boys of the royal family and to no one else.

They decided to visit Eklavya. When Dronacharya saw him, he remembered the boy.

Gazing upon Eklavya, Dronacharya felt wonder and amazement. The boy was clearly very talented, probably the most talented archer in the kingdom. That he considered him his guru and gave him credit for his accomplishments made Drona happy and proud. However, Drona was bound by the rules. There could be no greater warrior than the royal princes. As part of the royal entourage, Drona also understood the necessity of such a rule. After much thought, he found a solution to the dilemma.

'Eklavya, if you consider me your guru, then you owe me guru *dakshina*.'

'Ask anything of me, Dronacharya, for I am forever indebted to you. Had it not been for you, I wouldn't have been able to save the deer in the forest from all the leopards.'

'Give me your thumb.'

Arjuna and his brothers gasped; they couldn't believe their ears. They stood frozen and horrified as Eklavya, without a second thought, chopped his thumb off and presented it to his guru.

SIGNIFICANCE AND SYMBOLISM

The essence of childhood is innocence and a zest for life. On a physical level, the practice of yogasanas keeps our bodies spry and supple, like that of a child. Yogic breathing techniques and philosophy bring clarity to the minds and hearts of yogis, and this gives them an energy that is unique. In the practice of yoga, we try to retain a childlike and youthful wonder for life.

Yoga is also a means to remain fresh and inquisitive about ourselves. Far too often, we go about our lives mechanically, on auto mode. Our choices and decisions are made with little regard to what we actually want. We usually look outside for happiness and joy, and even for validation. However, we must look within for the answers we want. Just as the entire universe was in Krishna's mouth, we also have the wisdom of the universe within us. It is possible to tap into this wisdom with a little contemplation and meditation.

It is necessary to go inwards rather than outwards, and yoga is a means to do that.

When Yashoda saw the universe inside her child's mouth, it was symbolic of her role in the world. As a mother, her child was her universe and she was duty-bound to love and protect him. Even if it meant castigating him or punishing him for his errors, she would need to take the difficult path to carry out her responsibility as a mother.

When Eklavya was rejected by Dronacharya, he didn't lose courage, faith or hope. Nor was he bitter. He took it in his stride and didn't let it deter him from his goal.

Yoga is also a guru-shishya parampara and in such a relationship, we sometimes experience disappointment. The important thing is to continue learning and not lose faith in the guru.

Everyone encounters roadblocks and setbacks, but those who move forward with courage get closer to their goals than those who lose hope. The path of yoga keeps us moving forward with vigour and strength.

HOW TO

1.   Kneel on the floor with your feet and knees together.
2.   Sit back on your heels.
3.   Walk forward with your hands until your torso rests on your thighs. Place the forehead on the floor.
4.   Breathe.

HELPFUL HINTS

- Use a bolster/folded blanket under your hips if you're unable to sit on your heels. This variation also provides relief to tired legs.
- If your forehead doesn't touch the floor, use a block or a bolster under it.
- If you are pregnant, widen the knees while keeping your feet together and then bend forward. This will create space for your belly.

BENEFITS

- Cools the body and rests the mind.
- Stretches the shoulders, arms, chest and spine.
- Rests the lower body.
- Reduces menstrual pain.
- Massages the internal organs, particularly the digestive and reproductive organs, and keeps them healthy.
- Alleviates back pain.

CONTRAINDICATIONS

Because the joints of the lower body are used in this pose, practise with caution if you have an injury to the knee, ankles or hip joint.

4

trikonasana

(triangle pose)

Literally translated, *trikona* means three-sided.

    The trinity is perhaps the most recognized symbol in many cultures and religions. A trinity represents a fine balance. In an equilateral triangle, there are no weighted sides. The triangle exists in perfect balance because each vertex and side is perfectly equal to the others. The trinity of Brahma, Vishnu and Shiva represents birth, life and death. If any part of this trinity is absent or disturbed, the universe will cease to exist. The balance embodied by the trinity of Brahma–Vishnu–Shiva (which is required to sustain the universe), is represented by the *trikonasana*.

DISTRACTING THE GODS

Mahishasura was an evil buffalo demon. He was always up to some mischief. Mahishasura could morph into different shapes and sizes. He could not only control thoughts but also plant them into the minds of both devas and mortals. Although the devas were extremely troubled by him, they were powerless to control him. Aeons ago, he had been granted a boon that he could not be killed. Neither power nor reason prevailed over him.

Matters came to a head when one day, Mahishasura played a trick that offended everyone. He frequently disturbed the devas while they meditated, often putting an end to years of penance and austerities. This time, he decided to distract them by planting thoughts of sinful pleasures of the flesh in their minds. Everyone was puzzled and extremely embarrassed. When they found out that Mahishasura was the culprit, the devas joined forces against him. Surely, all their strength combined would be enough to overpower the devil. Many skirmishes later, however, they still hadn't found a solution to the problem.

'Something must be done about this,' Lord Vishnu said. 'This demon is getting more mischievous by the day. If we don't do something about it, he will soon be ruling the three worlds!'

Lord Brahma and Lord Shiva agreed. The three of them put their heads together and came up with a plan. They decided to create a goddess who was an illusion. Her name was Mahamaya, which means the 'great illusion'. Since she was only an illusion, Mahishasura's boon would be powerless against her. They also created a pet lion for her, who would help her slay the demon. Mahamaya and her lion engaged Mahishasura in a fierce battle. Everyone watched with bated breath. Mahamaya finally emerged victorious and everyone breathed a sigh of relief. All was well again in the three worlds.

A FINE BALANCE

For the world to exist as we know it, balance has to be maintained.

Brahma, Vishnu and Shiva were equally powerful. They had clearly defined responsibilities towards the universe and frequently got together to resolve problems. However, things are not always smooth even in the most cordial relationships, and friction rears its ugly head every once in a while.

One day, Vishnu and Brahma were resting. They were reminiscing about their past exploits. Invariably, the topic turned into a discussion about who was the more powerful of the two. They decided that whoever was more powerful deserved to be considered the leader.

'Creation is a magical thing,' asserted Lord Brahma. 'Whoever can create something out of nothing is endowed with true power. Therefore, we should agree that I am more powerful.'

'To ensure that everything that is created also endures is no mean feat,' responded Lord Vishnu. 'Ensuring harmony between different creatures requires great compassion and understanding. To ensure that creation endures is a work of great responsibility and power. I think I'm clearly the more powerful one and should be considered the leader.'

The argument between the two was threatening to become ugly. Hitherto, Lord Shiva had been only casually listening to the conversation. Now he felt he must intervene or the argument could have serious consequences.

Suddenly, a large pillar of raging fire appeared between Lord Vishnu and Lord Brahma. The pillar seemed to start in the heavens and go deep into the earth. Forgetting their argument, Lord Vishnu and Lord Brahma gazed at it with wonder and some anxiety. Then they decided to use the pillar to end their argument. The first one to find where the pillar originated or ended would be the leader.

'I will look for its origin,' declared Vishnu and dove down into the earth.

'I shall look for where it ends,' declared Brahma and flew heavenwards.

After some time, they met at the starting point again.

'Unfortunately, I couldn't find the origin of the pillar,' Vishnu confessed sadly.

'But I found the end!' Brahma lied gleefully. Shiva's anger flared up. Livid at Brahma's blatant lie, Shiva manifested himself. Both Vishnu and Brahma stared at him in amazement. Shiva calmly told them that the pillar of fire was a test.

'Vishnu, I'm happy that you remained honest. Brahma, if we are to work together for eternity, we must be honest with each other. Lying is unacceptable. I advise you both not to indulge in frivolous quarrels again.'

Saying this, Lord Shiva went back to his abode on Mount Kailash.

SIGNIFICANCE AND SYMBOLISM

Mahishasura represents all that makes us deviate from the path of goodness, integrity and honesty. Mahamaya represents the antithesis of Mahishasura. She stands for righteousness and fairness. Throughout our lives, there will be a tussle between the pull of temptation and the virtuous path. The trikonasana helps us find the fine balance between virtue and vice. This pose is about courage, precision and focus. Perhaps this is why Shiva's weapon of choice is the trident, a weapon symbolic of balance and strength.

The trikonasana depicts our past, present and future. When we hold this asana, these three phases of time converge in our limbs. To live a wholesome life, we must have a healthy acceptance of our past, be able to realistically gauge where we stand right now and feel optimistic about where we are going. When we practise acceptance of our past experiences, we can make the most of our present and build a brighter future. The back leg (representing the past) provides support needed to shape our present and consequently, our future. The front leg and arm reach out to the future. The hips and the placement thereof depict our present. When you reach forward into your future, do you do it with a clear disregard for and lack of thought about your past (physically embodied by the back leg), and which serves to ground you? Does your present support the future goals you have? To move into the future, we need an acceptance of the past and an understanding of the present.

The triangle represents stability, power, beauty and strength. It can maintain its shape without caving in to pressure on any side.

The ability to withstand pressure and the strength to retain its original shape are the qualities of a triangle, which we must meditate upon when we practise this pose. In the trikonasana, the yogi's mind, body and spirit (once again a trinity) become one.

HOW TO

1. Stand with your feet about four feet apart. The feet should be parallel to each other, toes pointing forward. Raise your arms, stretching your torso up from the waist.
2. Then stretch your arms out to shoulder level. Keep the neck long and shoulders relaxed.
3. Turn the right foot out so that the toes face away from the left foot. Extending from the hip, reach out to the right. Be careful not to lock your knees or hinge the hip.
4. Once you've stretched to your maximum, place your right hand on the floor, behind the right leg. Finally, extend the left hand.
5. Repeat on the left side.

HELPFUL HINTS

- If you are unable to reach the floor, rest your hand on yoga blocks.
- Taller practitioners can increase the distance between their feet to more than four feet.

BENEFITS

- Strengthens the legs and the knees.
- Opens up the chest, hip and groin region.
- Cultivates balance, both emotionally and physically.
- Tones and massages the abdominal organs.
- Provides relief from back pain and sciatica.

CONTRAINDICATIONS

The supported trikonasana (with props such as blocks) can be practised by anyone. It will prove beneficial to everyone. However, if you suffer from blood pressure problems, do not hold this pose for a long time. Similarly, if you have vertigo, practice only for short periods.

5

ardha chandrasana

(half moon pose)

Yoga is a practice of fullness, completeness and balance. It is interesting, then, that there are many 'half' poses in the practice.

CHURNING OF THE OCEAN

The devas and asuras looked intently at the Samudra Manthan, the churning of the great ocean in Hindu mythology. Everyone was waiting with bated breath for the amrit, the nectar of immortality. One after the other, many things emerged from the ocean, but the nectar was nowhere to be found. Everyone was caught unawares when a deadly poisonous mist, the *halahala*, appeared. It started to choke and poison the devas and the asuras alike, and very rapidly.

Only Lord Shiva was thought to be powerful enough to counter this horrific poison, and everyone looked to him for help. He was also quite puzzled. He had never come across a problem of this nature before and there was hardly any time to look for a solution.

Lord Shiva realized that the quickest thing to do would be to inhale the mist. Goddess Parvati, ever alert, was quick to react. She immediately clutched his neck and squeezed tight, preventing him from ingesting the poison and dying. However, the poison was so powerful that it burned Shiva's throat and skin even though Shiva had not swallowed even a drop of it. Everyone was alarmed as he started to turn blue.

Chandra, the moon, had been observing everything. He saw an opportunity to do his bit and help Lord Shiva. He came down and gently placed himself in Shiva's dreadlocks. This cooled Shiva down at once.

Even today, Lord Shiva is depicted with Chandra on his head. For this reason, Shiva is also called Chandrashekhara.

AN ANGRY MOON

The moon didn't always wax and wane.

Centuries ago, it would be full and resplendent in all its glory every night while Surya, the sun, took a break.

On one such bright, moonlit night, Ganesh was heading home from a feast. He was perched high on top of his ride, the mouse Krauncha. Both were making their way on the uneven, rocky roads. Fond of food and drink and all the other good things in life, Ganesh had overeaten. In the golden moonlight, Krauncha narrowly missed the snake that slithered across their path. He instinctively reared and Ganesh fell to the floor. His belly exploded and all the food he had consumed fell out. Undeterred, Ganesh picked up the food and put it back in his belly. Then he nonchalantly picked up the snake and tied it around his belly to keep the food safely in.

Chandra observed all this from his vantage point in the sky and couldn't help but laugh.

Ganesh, only a child, after all, felt insulted and threw one of his tusks at the moon, scarring him forever. But like the child he was, he wanted to cause more damage. He still felt enraged and wanted more vengeance. The only thing he could do was curse the moon. 'You are ugly and have a face that is scarred. Henceforth, you will stay hidden! And even if you appear and someone looks at you, it will bring them bad luck!' thundered a livid Ganesh.

Chandra was hurt and dejected, but powerless in the face of such a strong curse.

From then on, only Surya could appear. Because of the heat and the bright light that Surya brought, the plants started dying and the water dried up. There was no respite for animals or people and the entire ecosystem started to suffer. In addition to this, people couldn't sleep because of the bright sunlight. Their work and other duties were neglected. The love between human beings decreased as people became tired, restless, irritable and even ill.

Seeing the world in such distress, the gods held an emergency meeting. It was agreed that Ganesh should revoke his curse for the greater good. Ganesh was summoned.

After much discussion, cajoling and explaining, Ganesh agreed. But alas, he found that he didn't have the power to revoke the curse! Try as he might, he was unable to do it. The gods asked him to modify the curse since it appeared impossible to revoke.

Ganesh thought deeply. 'Chandra, from now on, you will appear only so that Surya can rest. But you won't be able to shine in all your glory.'

Chandra (like everyone else) was confused. Ganesh's words were unclear.

Ganesh explained further. 'Each night, you will decrease in size until you disappear. You won't be allowed to come out for an entire night. Then you'll start to increase in size until you reach your full size. But only for a day, and only one day in a month. In fact, the night you're gone will be considered holy. *And*, because you've offended me, you won't be allowed to come out during Ganesh Chaturthi!'

Finally, Ganesh felt satisfied. Not only had he punished the moon, he had also ensured that everyone would remember the slight done to him by Chandra.

The moon was sad, but was unable to do anything about it. He reconciled himself to thinking that it could've been much worse.

SIGNIFICANCE AND SYMBOLISM

This story illustrates that balance is integral. The sun and the moon are both important for all life and for our universe to continue. The world went into a tizzy when only the sun shone. As human beings, we are a balance of light and dark, and both are equally important for us to thrive. Instability occurs when one aspect starts to dominate. Along with the good times, it is necessary to accept the bad times. To experience gratitude, we need to be down in the dumps every once in a while.

For us to thrive just like the earth is thriving, we need to glean wisdom from the bad times. Then we need to use the power of this wisdom when we feel things are going smoothly for us.

Yoga seeks to teach the practitioner to appreciate what exists. As beautiful as the bright, full moon is, the delicate sliver of the moon towards the end of its cycle is also beautiful.

Rather than living in the past or in the perceived future, practitioners are encouraged to make peace with the present and to enjoy whatever it has to offer.

HOW TO

1. Start on the right with the trikonasana (Chapter 4).
2. Bend your right knee and reach forward with your right hand. Place it on the floor diagonally opposite the right foot.
3. Engage your right arm and leg, so that you can balance and support yourself on them. Slowly lift the left leg up until it is parallel to the floor or slightly above hip level.

4. To come down, bring your left leg back to the floor in the same way you took it up. You should end in the trikonasana again.

5. Repeat on the left side.

HELPFUL HINTS

- The extension of the torso is important. Your chest should be open and ribcage free. Both sides of your torso should be long and equal in length. Using a block to support your hand will enable you to lift and extend more effectively.

- Starting from the trikonasana and moving into the pose will help you understand the idea of transitioning between poses. This helps in finding balance when the external surroundings change, or when *we* may need to change to accommodate a new role, position or situation.

- Many practitioners like doing this pose against a wall. The wall gives you a 'safety net' should you lose your balance.

But there is nothing like learning how to trust yourself. Learning how to trust and have faith in yourself is the most valuable lesson of the half moon pose.

BENEFITS

- Strengthens the legs, spine and abdomen.
- Helps in reducing digestive problems, backache and sciatica.
- Great for stress relief.
- Improves balance and concentration.

CONTRAINDICATIONS

It's always a good idea to experiment with how you feel and how much your body is capable of on any given day. The ardha chandrasana requires a lot of awareness and balance and therefore, it should not be performed if you have a migraine or a headache. Also, never practice if your blood pressure has been unstable. Don't practice this pose if you've been ill, or have been suffering from diarrhoea, as it engages the abdominal muscles.

6

ardha matsyendrasana

(half lord of the fish pose)

You would think that the 'Lord of the Fish' would be a fish himself. But it's not so! There are references to Matsyendra in mythology, and also research showing that Matsyendra was, in fact, a man born in Bengal sometime around the tenth century. Unfortunately, there's not much else known about him.

THE SAGE WHO WASN'T A FISH

Once, there was a couple who had a child born at an inauspicious time. It was a commonly held belief that a child who'd had an untimely birth was an ill omen and would bring bad luck to the parents and the entire clan. Rather than risk bad luck, the parents decided to get rid of the infant. The next day, they threw him in the river. Little did they know that this child, who later came to be known as Matsyendra, would become one of the greatest sages of all time.

A giant fish swallowed Matsyendra whole and he lived inside the fish's belly for a long time. He grew up hale, hearty and happy.

One day, Shiva and Parvati were sitting on the banks of a river, talking to each other. After years of tapas and meditation, Lord Shiva had become enlightened about the practice of yoga. He came down from Mount Kailash specially to teach his consort Parvati the secrets of the great practice. As luck would have it, the giant fish happened to be swimming near the riverbank where Shiva and Parvati were sitting. Matsyendra was close by (in the fish's belly), listening to all the esoteric knowledge Shiva was imparting.

The fish was remarkably large, and when Parvati noticed it, she told Shiva. 'Who are you?' Shiva asked the fish. 'And why have you been swimming near us for so long? Why don't you go on your way?'

To their surprise, they heard a voice coming from the fish. It said, 'O Lord Shiva, the knowledge that you are imparting to Parvati interests me a great deal. I am mesmerized and unable to tear myself away from your words.'

Unable to contain his surprise, and impressed by these sentiments, Shiva asked the owner of the voice to reveal himself.

Matsyendra then narrated his entire ordeal, from how his parents abandoned him to how he grew up inside a fish and how fortunate he felt to be able to acquire the knowledge of yoga from Shiva himself. 'I know my parents considered me unlucky and inauspicious, my Lord, but with your blessings, I can be of good use to society,' said Matsyendra.

Touched, Shiva told Matsyendra that he was not unlucky. 'In fact, I choose you to take everything you've learned from me, and disseminate it to mankind.'

'It would be the greatest honour to do as you bid, my Lord,' said Matsyendra. 'But it is difficult to do that while inside a fish!'

Shiva at once transformed the giant fish into a man. This man came to be known as Matsyendranath, which means Lord of the Fish. Just like Shiva had commanded him to, he went on to teach yoga far and wide. In the yogic tradition, students go on to teach their own students, who further teach more students. Hence, it is believed that all modern yoga knowledge originates from Shiva and has been passed down to Matsyendranath and those who learnt from him.

One day, Matsyendranath decided that there was a need to collate all his knowledge of yoga and put it together for future generations. His compilations on yoga practice and philosophy comprise some of the earliest known texts on Hatha yoga. Centuries later, one of his descendants (Swatmarama) would write the *Hatha Yoga Pradipika* (see 'What Is Yoga?'). Yogis who study in the direct lineage of Matsyendranath are considered his descendants and are known as the Nath yogis. They are a respected sect of yogis even today.

SIGNIFICANCE AND SYMBOLISM

Although Matsyendra was abandoned by his parents and spent his childhood deep in the belly of a fish, he thrived because he never believed he was unlucky. Instead of wallowing in sadness, he accepted his circumstances with dignity and fortitude. And when the opportunity presented itself, he emerged from inside the fish's belly and fulfilled his destiny.

Ardha matsyendrasana is a deep spinal twist. It is also a twist of the gut. When we say 'gut instinct' or 'I have a feeling', it refers to intuition. As human beings, we know what we want, what is good for us, and what is wrong. But sometimes, we lack the courage to act upon these instincts. In the way Matsyendra became Matsyendranath, we need to delve into our innermost feelings to become who we really are.

This pose is a measure of how flexible you are in your mind and body. It's important for there to be a balance between the two. Those with very flexible bodies and spines have a tendency to twist out of proportion and injure themselves—or end up compromising so much in life that it leaves them exhausted and even harmed.

Similarly, the spine is a metaphor for courage and resilience. Words such as 'spineless' and 'no backbone' are derogatory. Our spines hold us up and a straight spine is a sign of a strong and confident personality. A hyper-flexible body seems almost 'spineless' and indicates greater vulnerability. Conversely, a rigid spine and being intractable leave little room for one to grow and learn in life. This pose is therapeutic for people who are tightly 'wound up' because of past trauma.

When practising this pose, we must find a balance between how much we want to do, how much we think we can do and how much we actually *can* do with correct alignment. At a deeper level, practitioners must ask themselves—how flexible do I want to be in my body and in my life? More flexible is not always better.

Done with some reflection, this pose helps yogis discover blocks in their bodies and in their lives. You will be able to look at your present and future without the fog of the past clouding your vision. You will experience clearer vision and perception.

HOW TO

1. Sit on the floor with your legs extended and your toes pointing up. Engage your core to keep the back of the knees pushed down. The torso must be perpendicular to the floor.
2. Bending the right leg, place the right foot on the outside of the left knee.
3. Bend the left leg so that the left foot sits next to the right buttock.
4. Twist your torso to the right.
5. Place the left elbow on the outside of the right knee and straighten the arm.
6. Place the left hand on the left knee.
7. Exhale and deepen your twist.
8. Look over your right shoulder.
9. Repeat on the left side.

HELPFUL HINTS

◈ If the above is too much for you, stop at Step 4. As your practice deepens, you'll be able to continue to the next step.

- It is a common tendency to hunch the back in Step 5. Avoid doing this. Keep the chest open and lengthen the spine upwards to create space between the vertebrae.

BENEFITS

- Stimulates your digestive system.
- Stretches the shoulders, chest, arms and spine.
- Reduces lower back ache.
- Trims the excess fat from the sides.
- Helps us realize that everything that has been 'twisted' can be untwisted.

CONTRAINDICATIONS

If you're injured, you should wait and heal before you start spine twisting asanas. The ardha matsyendrasana is a deep twist for your abdomen and spine. For this reason, you must be careful if you have stomach ulcers. Don't practice the pose if you've had recent abdominal surgery. Your shoulders and arms also play an important role in this asana, so perform it with caution if these are injured.

7

kurmasana

(tortoise pose)

There are repeated references to turtles in popular culture. The most famous story featuring these reptiles is perhaps that of the hare and the tortoise. This story teaches children the virtue of steadiness and perseverance versus the thrill of speed and rashness. Sometimes, it may seem like other people are ahead of you in your career, studies or even asana practice. But in the end, the person who stays true and honest to the goal will triumph. There are many stories related to turtles and tortoises in the Hindu epics.

LIFTING UP THE WORLD

The devas were in a fix. A deadly curse had rendered them powerless. A misunderstanding between Lord Indra and the Sage Durvasa had transpired. Despite Lord Indra repeatedly begging for forgiveness, Sage Durvasa remained adamant and would not retract or soften the curse.

The devas had lost their immortality, strength and divine powers. The kingdom of heaven was no longer theirs and the asuras troubled and harassed them daily. If this continued, they would perish and the universe would be doomed.

The devas knew they needed help. They decided to ask Lord Vishnu for guidance. They trusted him as he was understanding and wise.

'O Lord Vishnu!' they cried. 'As you know, we are being tormented by the asuras and unable to defend ourselves. We've come to you with hopes of an effective solution.'

Lord Vishnu was perplexed. 'It's Sage Durvasa who has cursed you,' he said. 'He is powerful and so are his curses. If you hope to counter his curse, you need something equally powerful. This situation is unprecedented. Give me some time to think.'

Saying this, Lord Vishnu began thinking deeply. He deliberated long and hard. Finally, he had an idea.

'If you drink the nectar of immortality, you will be able to counter Durvasa's horrible curse. But the nectar isn't easy to obtain. It lies at the bottom of the ocean and it will take great efforts to bring it up.'

The devas were undeterred by Lord Vishnu's warning. After much deliberation they came up with what they felt was a foolproof strategy.

The devas put into motion one of the largest group efforts the universe had ever seen. They enlisted the asuras and Vasuki the serpent to help them. Mount Mandara also volunteered and the great churning of the ocean for the nectar of immortality started.

However, once the churning started, Mount Mandara started sinking into the ocean! He was unable to withstand the force being used. Alarmed, everyone approached Lord Vishnu again. Vishnu, realizing the gravity of the situation and knowing there was very little time, morphed into a tortoise, or a *kurma*, and crawled under Mount Mandara to prevent it from sinking.

And so the churning continued.

THE SAGE WITH THE MANY WIVES

One of the first and most powerful sages of the Hindu pantheon was Sage Kashyap. *Kashyap* is also the Sanskrit word for turtle. Many hymns and verses in the Rig Veda are attributed to him. He was also one of the *saptarishis*, the rishis that were born from the mind of Brahma, and therefore highly revered. Sage Kashyap spent his time studying the Vedas and other religious texts and acquired a great amount of wisdom and knowledge.

King Daksha, the son of Lord Brahma, admired the sage and wished for him to marry all of his thirteen daughters. 'Sage Kashyap, you are honoured and revered, righteous and learned. It would be a great honour for me if you took all my daughters as your wives. I can't hope for a better husband for them.'

Sage Kashyap was in a fix. Although honoured by King Daksha's kind words, he didn't know if having multiple wives was allowed in the Vedas. But he had also agreed to help Lord Brahma create the universe by helping to populate the world. He could do this by fathering many children from his many wives.

It was decided he would marry all of King Daksha's daughters. Sage Kashyap's descendants went on to become eminent personalities in their times and thus, Sage Kashyap became the father of some noteworthy personalities in the Hindu pantheon.

SIGNIFICANCE AND SYMBOLISM

The tortoise can be compared to the sun. Both move very slowly, and never deviate from their path. They never get lost, always remain focused and rest periodically so that they can continue with the same intensity. The Samudra Manthan was a carefully thought-out plan, but when obstructions emerged, Lord Vishnu morphed into a tortoise to save the day. Instead of despairing, Lord Vishnu kept the goal in mind and, like a tortoise, continued towards it slowly and steadily.

The sun withdraws to rest as the moon rises and shines.

The tortoise withdraws into its shell to rest. Similarly, we need to recoup and rejuvenate at regular intervals to live life to our fullest potential.

It is important to consider this when we practise the *kurmasana*.

Although this pose initially makes practitioners feel claustrophobic and breathless, practising the kurmasana inculcates a sense of peace over time. You are sprawled face forward, with your arms pinned under your 'shell' or legs, unable to move freely. The tortoise is in this position perennially, but doesn't get anxious. When faced with danger, the tortoise uses the shell, which seemingly traps it, to withdraw to safety (after all, running is not really an option.) When Sage Kashyap was confused about King Daksha's request, he could have reacted with haste. However, he sought the middle path so that he could remain true to his chosen path as well as honour Daksha's request.

It is important for human beings to recognize feelings of fear and vulnerability and resist the overwhelming temptation to run. Instead, we need to calmly assess the situation and decide on the best course of action to protect ourselves. Emotional security and freedom from anxiety come only by facing life instead of running from it.

The peace and calm that this pose brings also give us time and space to analyse our emotions. By understanding ourselves, we can take decisions that are best for our physical and mental well-being.

The imagery of the tortoise's shell is important. When faced with a dangerous situation, the kurma withdraws into its shell. Fear results in searching for protection. But these shells we run to, are they sturdy and strong? Or do they merely give the illusion of protection, comfort and safety? Are we drawing healthy boundaries or are we retreating into defensiveness, loneliness and self-sabotage? When a tortoise is on its back, it is helpless. Do our 'shells' only provide a facade of safety, or do they enable us to become stronger to face the challenges of life?

HOW TO

1.   Make sure your lower body is warmed up before practising this asana because it is an advanced asana.
2.   Sit with your legs about the distance of the mat apart.
3.   Bend your knees slightly and leaning your torso forward insert the arms under the knees and extend them outwards.
4.   Extend your trunk forward, creating space in the ribcage. Continue to extend the torso towards the floor. Extend your chin forward until the torso finally rests on the floor.
5.   Breathe deeply.

HELPFUL HINT

◉   Initially, rest your torso on a bolster. As your lower body becomes more flexible, you will be able to lower yourself to the floor.

BENEFITS

◉   Great to open up the lower body, particularly the hip joint.
◉   Alleviates lower back pain.
◉   Massages the abdominal organs.
◉   Alleviates symptoms of irregular and painful menstruation.

CONTRAINDICATIONS

As mentioned before, this is an advanced asana and should only be performed if your body is sufficiently warmed up. Don't practise it if you're recuperating from a hip injury. Since this pose requires the abdomen to be pushed to the floor, don't perform it if you are pregnant. Also avoid it if you have high blood pressure as this asana forces the blood to rush to the head.

garudasana
(page 46)

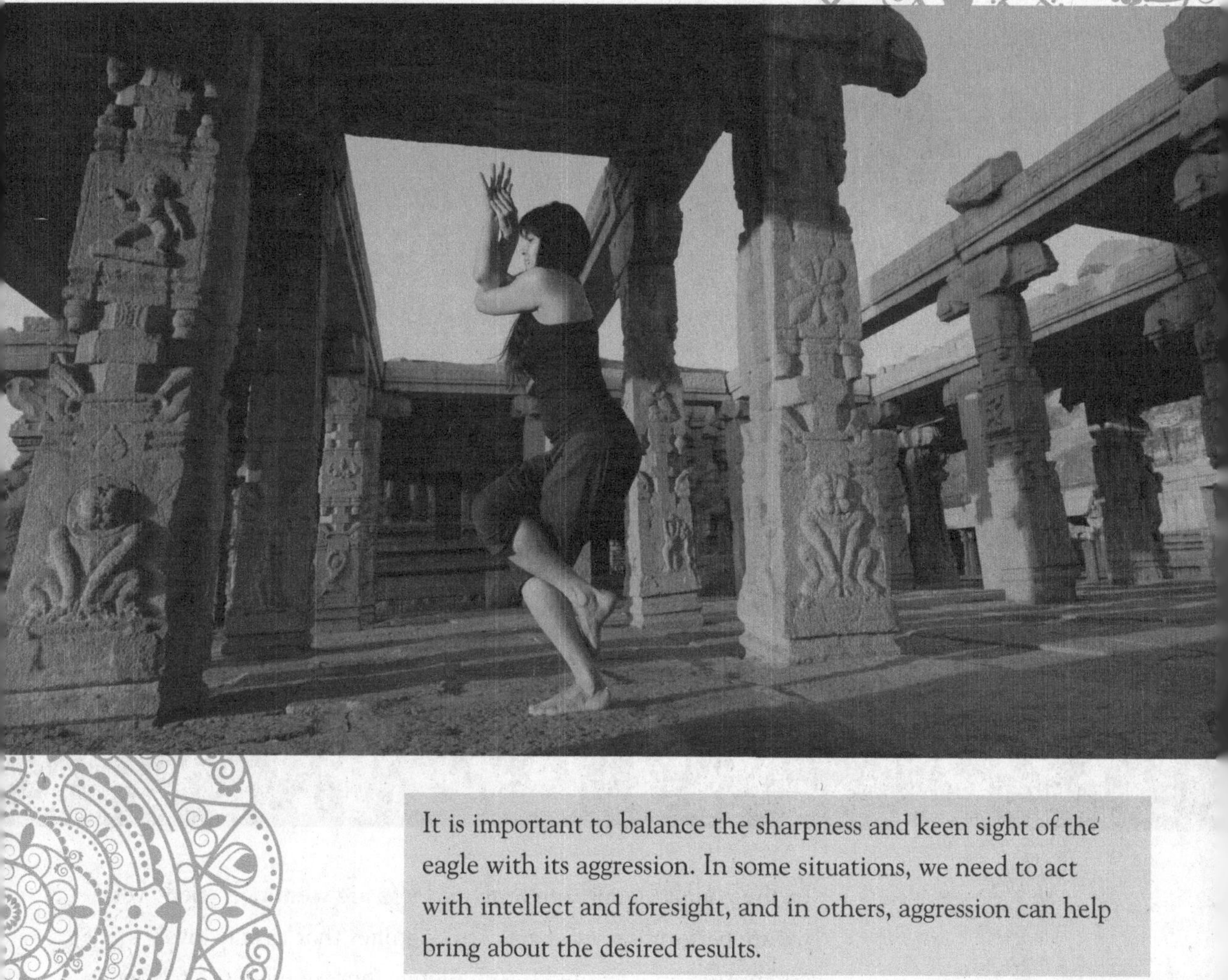

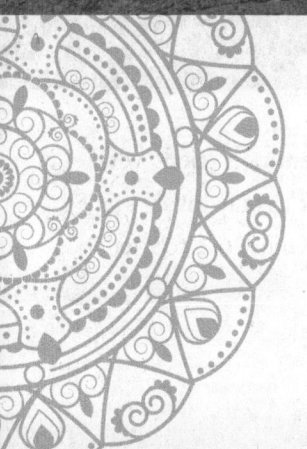

It is important to balance the sharpness and keen sight of the eagle with its aggression. In some situations, we need to act with intellect and foresight, and in others, aggression can help bring about the desired results.

gomukhasana
(page 51)

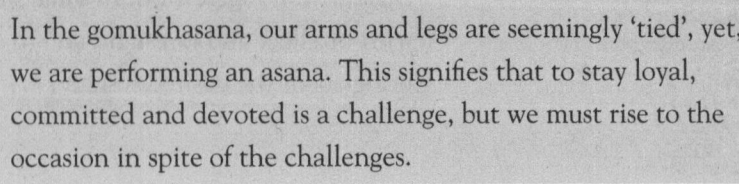

In the gomukhasana, our arms and legs are seemingly 'tied', yet, we are performing an asana. This signifies that to stay loyal, committed and devoted is a challenge, but we must rise to the occasion in spite of the challenges.

ashtavakrasana
(page 58)

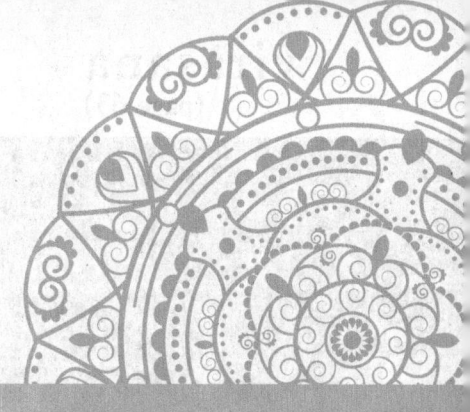

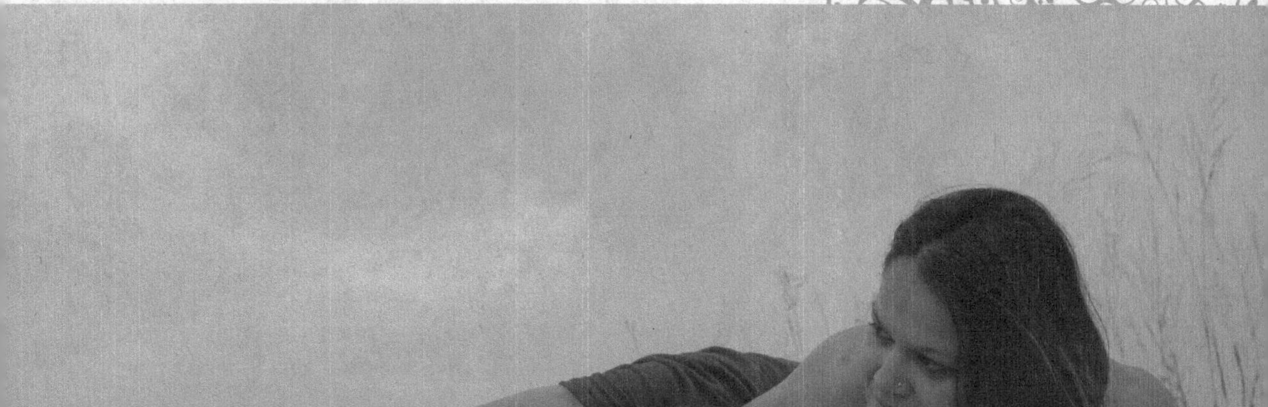

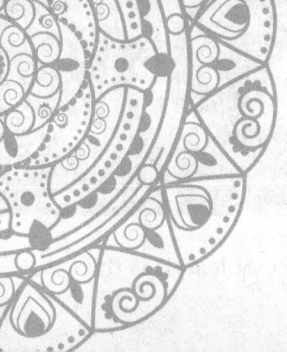

Ashtavakrasana is a reminder that yoga is not merely about the body, but also about the quest of the soul.

virasana
(page 63)

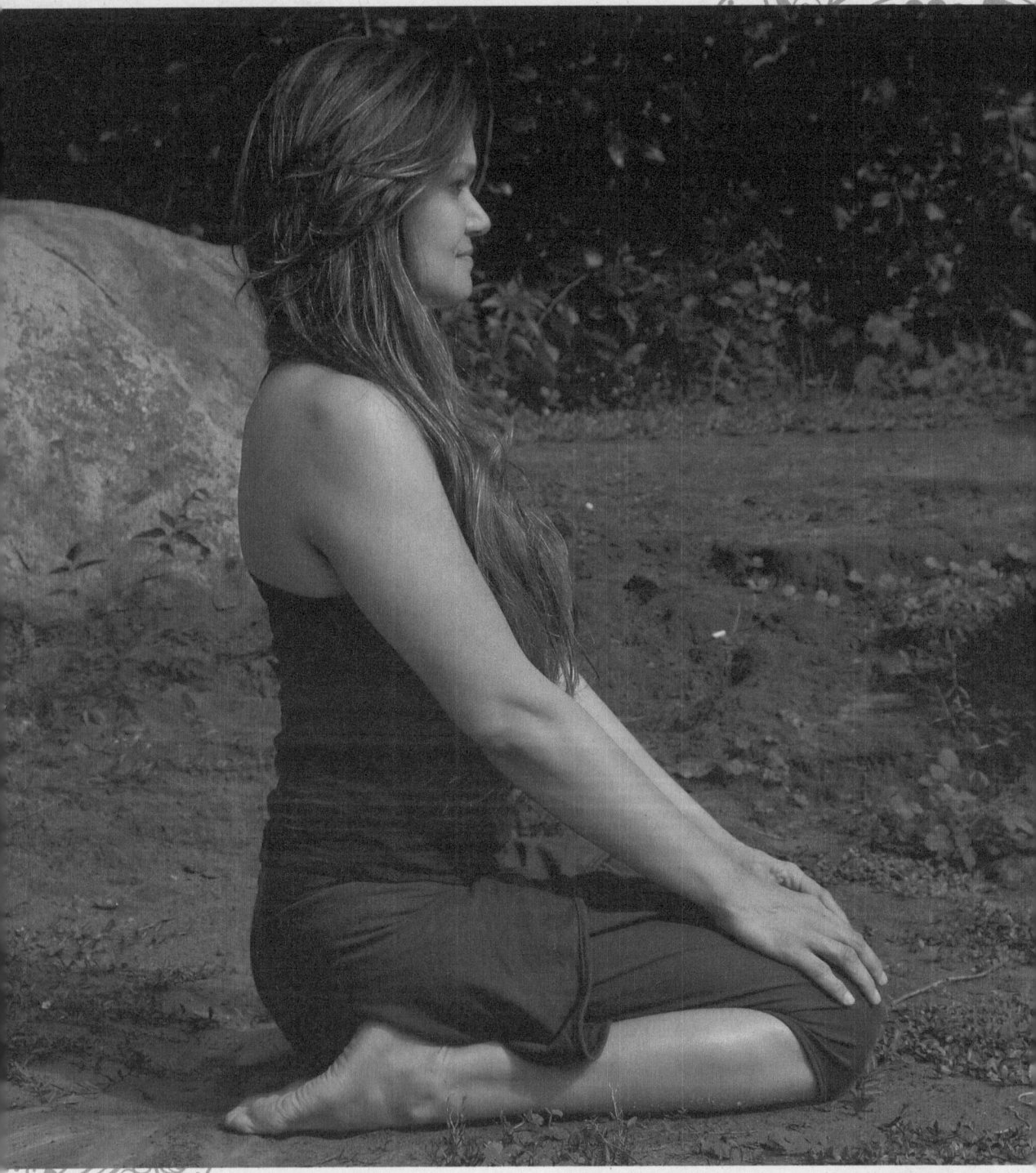

Bravery isn't the absence of fear, it is the mastery of fear.

marichyasana
(page 68)

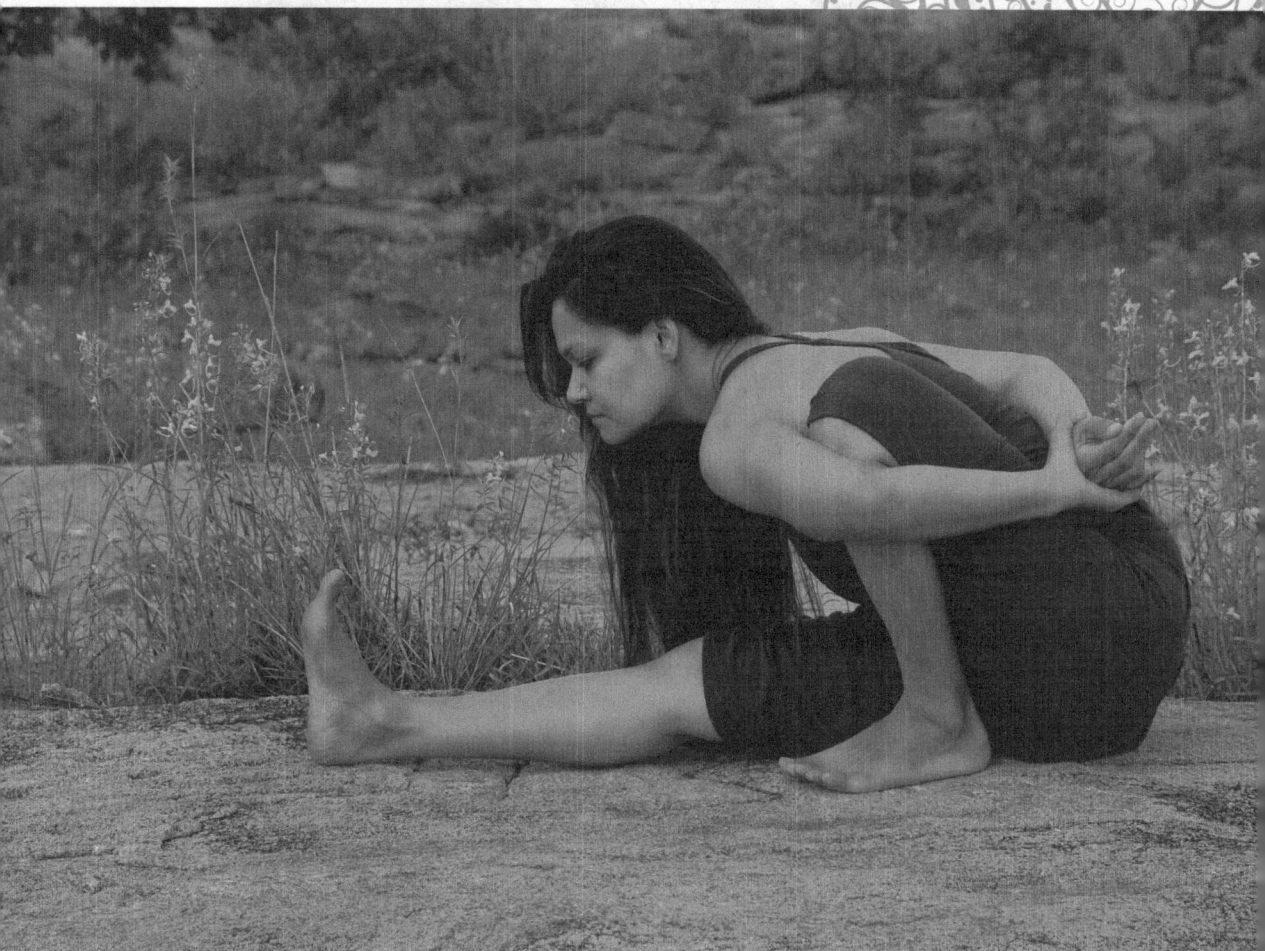

The challenge in life is to make the most of situations. The key to doing that is to persevere through seemingly unyielding circumstances.

padmasana
(page 73)

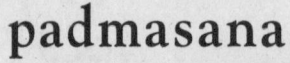

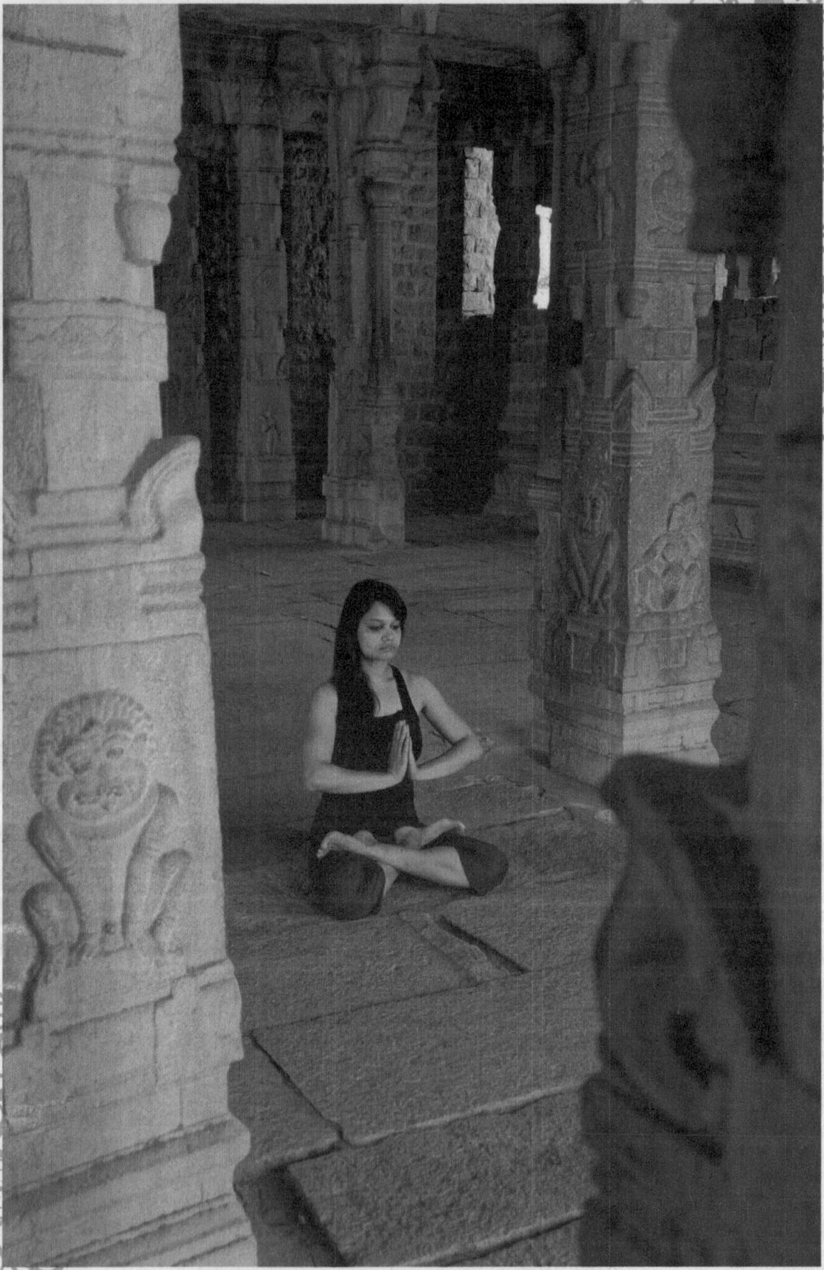

A lotus grows in muddy waters, but is never muddied. Similarly, we should be able to live in a world full of vices and temptations and yet stay focused on the purpose of our lives.

bharadwajasana
(page 77)

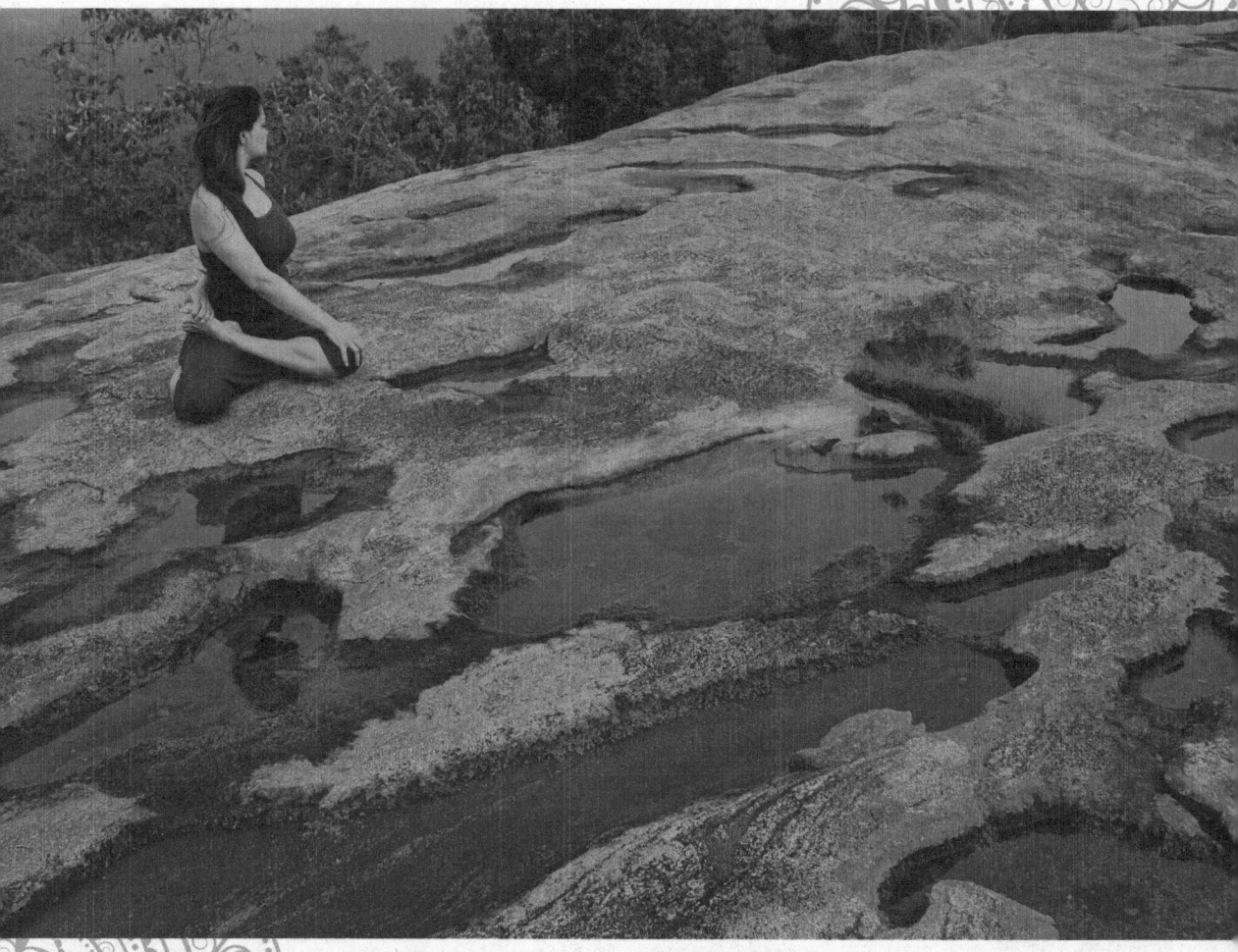

Once our thoughts are aligned, we must try to align our worlds. When there is alignment, there is a sense of balance. And that is the true purpose of yoga.

bhujangasana
(page 83)

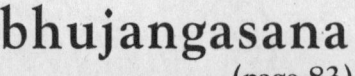

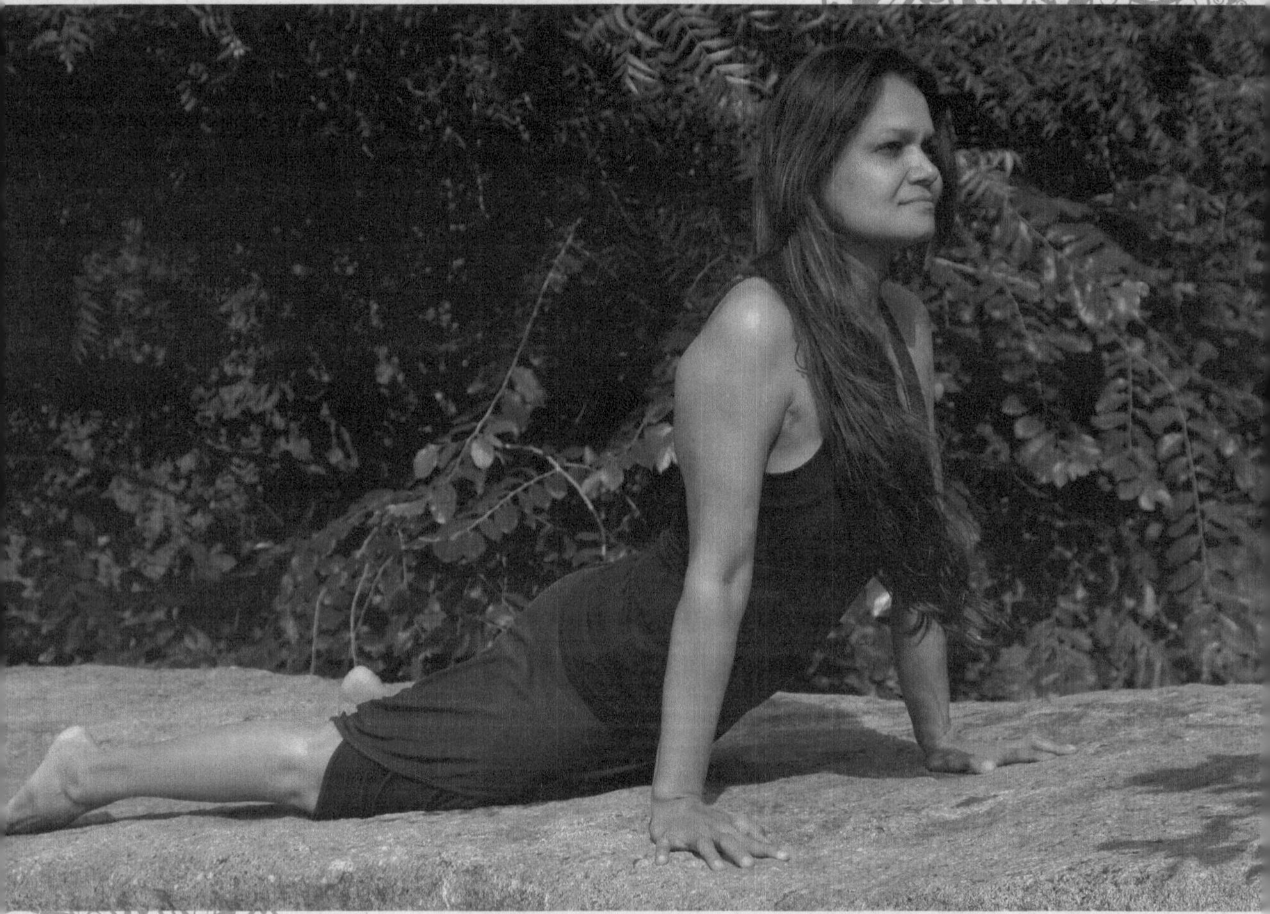

Life and situations require us to renew, rethink and reinvent ourselves. Growth can only happen if we shed the old and insignificant and walk towards the new.

8

tadasana

(mountain pose)

Mountains are significant in Hindu epics and mythology. The Himalayas have fascinated us for aeons and continue to do so even today. All the sacred rivers, such as the Ganges, originate from the mountains. It's little wonder, then, that mountains make their way into yoga folklore too, the most significant being Mount Kailash, the abode of Lord Shiva.

THE MOST MAGNIFICENT OF THEM ALL

King Himavat lived a quiet and pious life in his kingdom of snow. His kingdom was formidable and intimidating. It was as vast as it was cold. He lived there with his consort, Queen Mena, the daughter of Mount Meru.

King Himavat maintained a peaceful kingdom. It flourished under his benign rule. There was no fighting or danger. His subjects spent their time in prayer and austerities. King Himavat was responsible, kind and charitable.

He had three daughters and a son with his queen. Each of his daughters was blessed with a different personality. Ragini was fair and had a rosy complexion. She was delicate and kind and preferred red clothing. Kutila was fair and wore flowers around her neck. She preferred the colour white. The last daughter was Kali, who was as dark as the night.

In the true ethos of the kingdom, the daughters were encouraged to meditate, pray and practise devotion and austerities. Ragini, Kutila and Kali were all enamoured by Lord Shiva. Each prayed that her future husband be as powerful and virtuous as Lord Shiva, if not Shiva himself.

Finally, Kutila's prayers were heard. She would marry Lord Shiva!

Lord Brahma saw all that was happening with some alarm. He immediately manifested himself and intervened. 'Kutila has undoubtedly been earnest and devoted in her prayers. But someone as delicate as our dear Kutila will not be able to bear a son for Shiva!'

Kutila was devastated. This was her only wish in life and all she had ever prayed for. She felt it was being unfairly denied to her. She knew she could bear sons for Shiva, and told Brahma so.

Lord Brahma shook his head sadly and said, 'I understand you are dejected, Kutila, but someone as delicate and fair as you is not suited for Shiva.'

'How can you say that, Lord Brahma?' cried Kutila defiantly. 'Who knows the future? I'm sure I will be able to bear strong and healthy sons for Shiva.'

Brahma, already a tad impatient, was furious at her insouciance and cursed her to become a river in her father's kingdom.

After some time, Ragini's prayers were heard. Once again, Lord Brahma appeared.

'Ragini, you too, like your sister, won't be able to bear Shiva a son,' he declared regretfully.

Mena watched the exchange between them with some trepidation. She was still coming to terms with the loss of one daughter. Mena cautioned Ragini not to offend

Lord Brahma in any way. Ragini wanted to heed her mother's advice, but the pain of rejection was too great. 'How can it be that neither my sister nor I can provide a son to Lord Shiva?' she argued indignantly. 'Kutila may have been fair and delicate, but I'm strong and healthy!'

Lord Brahma shook his head sadly again. 'You may feel that you are strong, dear Ragini. But Shiva needs someone stronger to bear his sons.'

Like Kutila, Ragini continued to argue.

Brahma's deadly anger flared up once again. 'Just as I cursed your sister, I shall curse you too, Ragini. You will never leave your father's kingdom. You will become the soft evening light that falls daily and is admired by everyone. You will always remain fair and beautiful and lovely. Maybe Shiva himself will admire you, but you will never become his wife!'

Finally, it was Kali's turn. Having already lost two daughters, Mena was beside herself with anxiety.

'O daughter!' she cried. 'I'm yet to get over the pain and grief of losing your sisters. It fills me with unimaginable dread to think of losing you too. Put Lord Shiva out of your mind. We shall get you a better husband!'

Kali, however, was excited. Shiva was already hers in her mind and she was looking forward to meeting him in the flesh. She dismissed her mother's entreaties as maternal concern and continued to pray for Lord Shiva.

Finally, Lord Brahma came to see Himavat's third daughter. As his gaze fell on her, he smiled broadly.

'O Kali, your powerful limbs and strong disposition are perfect for bearing many strong, healthy and powerful sons for Shiva!'

King Himavat had been a silent observer of his daughters' fates. Although Kali finally got what she desired, he was disappointed. Himavat knew Shiva was a homeless mendicant and wanderer. As he looked at his vast kingdom, he wondered if Shiva would be able to provide Kali the comforts she was used to.

But Kali was ecstatic and Mena was already planning a grand wedding. King Himavat reluctantly went along with the marriage. In the years to come, he would constantly test Shiva. As a father, he needed reassurance that his daughter was happy. Shiva understood his sentiments. Over the years, Shiva gained Himavat's trust. King Himavat saw that Kali and Shiva complemented each other beautifully. While he was silent, she was dynamic. Both lived together through the aeons beautifully. Eventually, King Himavat came to respect Lord Shiva and his abode in Mount Kailash.

SIGNIFICANCE AND SYMBOLISM

Mountains signify challenges, which is why they are so intimately linked to yogis and yoga. The path of yoga is fraught with challenges. Making time to practice daily, inculcating the yamas and niyamas into routine life and living by the tenets of yoga are tough challenges. It is easy to lose track of ourselves and the practice, but with consistent discipline and hard work, it is possible to remain focused.

As yoga practitioners, we need to be like the great mountains—rooted to the ground, yet reaching up to the heavens. Challenges need to be overcome with courage, resolve and good emotional and physical health.

Summitting a mountain is a big achievement. From the peak of the mountain, everything looks minuscule and insignificant. When we achieve our goals, the problems that we were initially worried about seem insignificant and petty. As you diligently work towards a goal, your problems will melt away and seem less daunting. It is no wonder, then, that we retreat to the mountains to gain insight, wisdom and new perspective.

The *tadasana* is also called *samasthiti*, which means straight, upright and steady. All yogasanas start and end with the samasthiti.

Before any movement, there has to be stillness, stability and balance. This pose calls for us to be steady and strong like a mountain.

HOW TO

1. Stand with your feet together, their inner edges touching. Distribute your weight evenly on the soles of your feet. Your neck should be erect but relaxed.
2. Elevate your chest and relax your shoulders.
3. Reach down with your arms along the sides of your body, as though you're reaching for the floor. The palms should be turned in towards your body.
4. Tighten the kneecaps.
5. Keep your gaze focused but relaxed.

HELPFUL HINT

*   Stand with your feet about four inches apart if you're unable to balance with the feet together.

BENEFITS

*   Improves posture and balance.
*   Helps alleviate symptoms of flat feet.
*   Strengthens the legs.

CONTRAINDICATIONS

Anyone can practise the tadasana!

9

garudasana

(eagle pose)

Yoga philosophy postulates an interconnection between living things. All living things are considered equal and we see them all play important roles in mythology. Birds, particularly, have demonstrated loyalty, fealty and compassion time and time again.

SAVING THE DAY

When the devas and asuras churned the ocean for the nectar of immortality, the snakes decided they also wanted some of the amrit. But they had neither the strength nor the courage to get it by themselves. So they hatched a devious scheme. They would kidnap Vinata, Garuda's mother, and hold her ransom. Then they would make Garuda do their bidding.

Garuda was the vehicle of Lord Vishnu and the king of birds. He was part man, part eagle. He had the head and wings of an eagle and the body of a man. He had hatched from a huge egg and was radiant. It is said that he shone with the light of a million suns. In fact, the gods asked him to dim his radiance a little because it was blinding everyone. Garuda had the strength, foresight and intellect of an eagle.

When he found that his mother had been kidnapped for ransom, he seethed with rage. Garuda knew that he would need his brute strength and intellect to rescue her. The snakes told Garuda that they would exchange his mother for some amrit. The amrit was on a high mountain and the snakes couldn't slither to the top. But Garuda could easily fly to the summit.

Although Garuda could soar to the top, there were many dangerous obstacles along the way he did not anticipate.

The first obstacle was a ring of fire, which he had to fly through. Garuda knew that if his wings got singed, then he wouldn't be able to continue flying. Perhaps, if he was very careful, then he could avoid getting his wings burned. Finally, he decided that rather than taking a chance, he would douse the fire with water from a nearby river.

Next, he encountered a circular door which had spiked metal rings rotating in opposite directions. Garuda reduced himself to the size of a fly and flew through the door.

His final obstacle were two poisonous snakes. They were fierce, angry and lethal. Garuda decided to first startle them by flapping his wings vigorously. They were caught off-guard and before they could recover, he used his strong, sharp beak to kill them. Since then, snakes have been afraid of eagles.

Finally, he found the amrit and flew back with it.

The gods had been observing everything and they knew the snakes holding Garuda's mother ransom would misuse the powers the amrit would give them. So, just as the snakes were about to drink the amrit, the gods intervened. Even then, the snakes managed to consume two drops. The amrit was so potent that those drops painfully split their tongues in two—hence the fork on the sinister tongues of snakes.

THE GREAT GOOD BIRD

One day, Jatayu, the good eagle, was flying around the beautiful forest. He was smiling to himself as he admired the flora and the fauna. Everything was peaceful, fragrant and calm.

Suddenly, a horrific scream pierced the silence. It caused the leaves to rustle unexpectedly and startled the birds. The smaller birds flew away in fear, but Jatayu was curious and concerned. He immediately flew towards the direction of the screams. Perhaps someone needed help.

He followed the screams and came upon Ravana's *vimana*. He saw Sita struggling in Ravana's ruthless grip and understood what was happening. He flew towards Ravana, intending to free Sita by pecking Ravana painfully. A great tussle ensued. Finally, Ravana, fearsome and powerful, managed to hack off Jatayu's wings and he fell to the ground, writhing in pain.

Jatayu knew he was dying. He had been a great devotee of Lord Rama throughout his life and wanted to be of service to him before he died. He knew that Lord Rama and his brother Lakshmana would be searching for Sita, and would sooner or later find him. Although in great pain, he kept breathing laboriously. When Rama and Lakshmana finally found him, he narrated the events to them with every ounce of his remaining energy.

Rama and Lakshmana expressed their deep gratitude to Jatayu.

'I have one final request, O Lord,' Jatayu whimpered to Rama. 'Please end my misery with your own two hands. It would be a blessing and an honour to attain mukti at your hands, O Lord!'

Rama, ever compassionate and kind, and a strict follower of dharma, understood. With one swift and powerful blow, he ended Jatayu's suffering. As they stood over the now lifeless bird, Rama and Lakshmana felt a great sorrow. They had always had great regard for Jatayu and honoured him by conducting his funeral rites as they would of a member of their own family.

SIGNIFICANCE AND SYMBOLISM

The eagle has power, sharpness, agility, speed and great eyesight. It is feared by its prey. From its high vantage point, it can surreptitiously observe its prey and swoop in for the kill.

Though Garuda and Jatayu are both winged creatures reminiscent of the eagle, they represent different aspects of the bird.

When we practice the *garudasana*, we need to meditate upon Garuda's bravery, his courage and his laser-sharp focus. When faced with challenges in life, these are the skills that will see us through.

Jatayu's devotion is unparalleled. As soon as he saw Sita needed help, he rose to the occasion. Even though Ravana repeatedly wounded him, and he knew that he could be fatally wounded, Jatayu continued to fight. Later, even in the throes of pain, he wanted to be of help.

The eagle is also an aggressive bird. A negative emotion such as aggression can hinder a situation.

It is important to balance the sharpness and keen sight of the eagle with its aggression. In some situations, we need to act with intellect and foresight, and in others, aggression can help bring about the desired results.

HOW TO

1. Stand in tadasana (see Chapter 8).
2. Cross the right leg over the left. Go further and hook the left foot behind the right calf.
3. Wrap the right arm around the left.
4. Repeat on the other side.

BENEFITS

- Strengthens the legs, arms, shoulders and wrists.

- Stretches the hips.
- Great to treat backache and sciatica.
- Improves balance and concentration.

CONTRAINDICATIONS

Although the garudasana is a balancing asana, it is also a deep stretch for the ankles and knees. If you've injured the joints of the lower body, then wait to heal before you start practising this asana. Avoid if you are suffering from vertigo and migraines.

10

gomukhasana

(cow-faced pose)

The cow plays a significant role in Indian culture, literature and tradition. Indian mythology considers cows sacred. The cow is referred to as '*gau mata*' or 'mother cow'. Cows are worshipped as a symbol of motherhood. Their milk is used to make butter and ghee and even their urine and dung are used for therapeutic and healing purposes. The following stories illustrate why cows hold such a special place in mythology.

DEVOTION, LOYALTY AND A LONG LIFE

Sage Shilada was a great devotee of Lord Shiva. He had been yearning for a child for years, but his desire remained unfulfilled. Many people proposed solutions, but nothing worked. Finally, he decided to perform intense penance to Lord Shiva. He knew it was difficult to please Shiva, but he was willing to go to great lengths. He performed many austerities and left no stone unturned. At last, Lord Shiva was satisfied and appeared before Shilada.

'Shilada, your hard work and sacrifices make me very happy. I am moved by your devotion. I have decided to grant you your wish. Tell me, what do you wish for?'

Shilada's joy knew no bounds. It was hard for him to believe that his years of penance had finally borne fruit. 'For as long as I can remember, I've wished only for a child, my Lord,' said Shilada. 'I wish for a child I can call my own, to hold, to love and to cherish.'

'So it shall be,' Shiva declared and disappeared.

The next day, while Shilada was ploughing his land, he found a beautiful baby boy.

Shiva's voice boomed suddenly, 'Shilada, I have granted your wish! Take the child. Bring him up well.'

Shilada was overjoyed and took the baby home. He named the boy Nandi. Under Shilada's care and guidance, Nandi grew up to be a handsome, responsible and good boy. Unsurprisingly, he was also a great devotee of Lord Shiva.

One day, two sages, Mitra and Varuna, came to their house.

'Nandi, these sages are highly learned, respected and revered,' Shilada said. 'Please take care of them and ensure they are comfortable.'

All went well and it was finally time for the sages to leave. As was the custom, both Shilada and Nandi asked them for their blessings. The sages smiled benevolently and blessed Shilada. But when it was time to bless Nandi, their smiles faded and they looked at each other hesitantly.

Nandi was confused and Shilada was filled with foreboding. 'O great sages! Why this hesitation in blessing my good son?' he asked.

Mitra and Varuna looked at each other sadly. Both seemed reluctant to speak. But Shilada was persistent and they finally had to tell him. 'Forgive us, Shilada,' they said. 'We don't want to be the bearers of bad news, but we have seen into the future. Your son Nandi will soon perish!' Shilada was dumbstruck and heartbroken.

Nandi was a devotee of Lord Shiva and had exceptional faith in him. Instead of wasting time in despair, he started praying to Lord Shiva. Pleased, Shiva appeared to him, just as he had appeared to his father years ago.

'I'm pleased by your penance, Nandi,' Shiva said to him. 'Tell me, is there something you want?'

'O Lord!' he cried. 'All this time, I thought I wanted a boon to live forever. But now, seeing you in front of me, the only desire I have is to serve you forever. Please Lord, keep me with you so that I can spend my days in service to you.' Saying this, he prostrated himself in front of Lord Shiva.

Shiva was happy with the intensity of Nandi's devotion and wanted to grant him his wish. Lord Shiva had just lost his beloved bull. The bull had been his constant companion, even keeping watch over his house as Lord Shiva slept.

'Nandi, there is a way that you can stay with me forever. I had a bull I loved dearly. He was with me all the time, a true friend to me. Since he passed away, I feel bereft and lonesome. Would you like to take his place?'

Nandi's joy knew no bounds. He agreed with great alacrity.

'But,' said Shiva, 'you will have to detach yourself from your earthly form, even taking on the face of a bull. You will also have to leave your father and stay with me in Mount Kailash.'

Nandi could hardly believe his ears. This was beyond anything he had imagined and he was excited. Lord Shiva was asking him to be his vehicle, his companion and his friend.

The devotion, affection and loyalty that Nandi felt for Lord Shiva was incomparable.

When the ocean was churned for the nectar of immortality, halahala, a deadly poison, emerged. It was so potent that it could wipe out the entire universe. Everyone was frightened and in despair, but Shiva volunteered to drink the poison and save the universe. Nandi watched horrified as his hero, lord and saviour drank the poison and held it in his throat.

So, when a bit of that poison fell on the earth, Nandi saved the day by quickly drinking it. Everyone stared in astonishment, but Nandi only smiled. He was an ardent devotee and knew that with Lord Shiva's grace, nothing would ever happen to him. Such was his faith.

KAMDHENU—BOVINE LOYALTY

The celestial cow Kamdhenu emerged from the churning of the ocean for the nectar of immortality. Kamdhenu means 'cow of plenty'. Whoever she belonged to would always be protected and have all their wishes granted. It was decided that Sage Vashishtha should keep her because sages needed cows' milk to make ghee for their pujas. Since then, Sage Vashishtha always had her protection and blessings.

One day, King Vishwamitra arrived in Sage Vashishtha's hermitage. As was the custom, the entire entourage was welcomed with a sumptuous meal. Everyone enjoyed the mouth-watering delicacies and ate heartily. King Vishwamitra was pleased but also surprised by the welcome.

'What a great meal we've had,' he told his men. 'Although hermitages are humble dwellings, Sage Vashishtha has arranged for such a lavish meal to welcome us. May he and his hermitage always be blessed and happy.'

'But my Lord,' spoke up one of his men, 'it is indeed no surprise that he is able to arrange such an opulent meal for us. Anyone in possession of a wish-granting cow such as Kamdhenu would be able to provide such a meal.'

King Vishwamitra was fascinated by the wish-granting cow. And the more he thought about Kamdhenu, the more he wanted to possess her. He decided to speak to Vashishtha about it.

'O Sage Vashishtha, I know your cow is precious to you, and useful too. However, ever since I've learned of her, I can't help but think that she can be useful for large armies such as mine. We travel and journey over great distances, and to have a cow that can constantly provide nourishment for our warriors would be a great blessing. O kind sage, please consider giving your cow to me. I will keep her happy and content. In return, I will give you whatever you want—any number of elephants, cattle, horses or even jewels!'

'It is kind of you to offer such wealth to me,' Sage Vashishtha told King Vishwamitra. 'But I can't do what you ask of me. Kamdhenu not only takes care of me and helps me in my day-to-day life, she is also a part of my family. Parting with her will leave me sorrowful and unhappy.'

King Vishwamitra could understand the sage's sentiments, but his desire for the cow exceeded his desire to be fair. He decided to take the cow by force. He rallied his army and captured Kamdhenu. Sage Vashishtha tried to protest and protect Kamdhenu, but he was powerless against the warriors.

Kamdhenu, ever ready to help Vashishtha, said to him, 'O Great Sage! Just command me, and I shall help you in defeating this army!'

Vashishtha did so, and Kamdhenu produced many valiant and strong soldiers who decimated King Vishwamitra's warriors.

King Vishwamitra had lost and needless to say, vowed revenge on Vashishtha. His revenge would take decades, but would be the most transformative experience of his life.

SIGNIFICANCE AND SYMBOLISM

Lord Krishna is called Gopala, which means 'protector of the cows' or 'the person who takes care of the cows'. There are numerous paintings and works of art that depict Shiva and Parvati with their children, riding Nandi, the bull. It sits outside all Shiva temples.

The practice of yoga is not one of quick results. When a practitioner decides to walk on the yogic path, it is with an understanding that the path of yoga spans lifetimes. Yogis must be willing to do their best in each life with the faith that with each lifetime, they are coming closer to samadhi, which is the final stage of the Ashtanga system of yoga. In this stage, the practitioner merges with the Infinite, the Eternal. This is the ultimate goal of yoga. The path to samadhi is a long and arduous one, fraught with challenges and difficulties. In the face of imminent defeat, both Kamdhenu and Nandi had the choice to give up and change the course of their lives. However, they persisted and eventually enjoyed the fruits of their labours. Just like Kamdhenu and Nandi, if yogis keep their dedication, faith and devotion securely in their hearts, they will experience samadhi, an existence devoid of any duality.

In the *gomukhasana*, our arms and legs are seemingly 'tied', yet, we are performing an asana. This signifies that to stay loyal, committed and devoted is a challenge, but we must rise to the occasion in spite of the challenges. When practising the gomukhasana, we must dwell on the loyalty and devotion Kamdhenu and Nandi had for their masters.

HOW TO

1. Sit with your legs extended out in front of you.
2. Bend your right leg and place the foot next to the left thigh.
3. Do the same on the left leg and align the knees on top of each other.
4. Reach up and back with your right arm.
5. Bend the left arm behind your back and grasp both hands together.
6. Repeat on the left side.

HELPFUL HINT

- Use a belt if you are unable to clasp your hands together behind your back.

BENEFITS

- Improves posture and breathing.
- Helps in releasing tension from the shoulders.
- Increases flexibility of the shoulder joints and the elbows.

CONTRAINDICATIONS

This is an intense stretch for the shoulders and upper back. Don't push yourself to do this asana if you have an injured shoulder, elbow, wrist, knee or ankle. This will only aggravate the injury.

11

ashtavakrasana

(eight-angle pose)

'Ashta' means eight. This pose is named after Ashtavakra, the sage whose body was bent at eight different places.

BENT OUT OF SHAPE

Once, there lived a great sage and his wife. The sage was proficient in the study of the Vedas and used to recite them daily. His wife was a good, dutiful wife and they lived together in marital bliss. They were soon going to have a child and were both very excited about it. Their child would be sage Ashtavakra, but they didn't know that yet.

When Ashtavakra was still in his mother's womb, he could hear everything that happened in the world, including his father's recitation of the Vedas. Although his father was very earnest in his recitations and an expert on the Vedas, he mispronounced many words.

Ashtavakra, who was destined to become a great sage, got irked every time he heard a mispronounced word. He felt that he should correct his father, but he also knew that this may be considered disrespectful. However, since his father recited the Vedas every day, he decided to take a chance and correct him. So great was Ashtavakra's divinity that he could speak in the womb and be heard by his parents.

All hell broke loose when he tried to rectify his father's recitation.

His father was livid and cursed him. The curse was so powerful that it caused his body to break in eight different places, although he was still in his mother's belly!

He was born deformed. His body never healed from the eight injuries and he was bent painfully at each one. His deformity was a source of great agony to his parents. His father saw the pain even the most mundane task caused Ashtavakra and regretted having lost his temper. There was no way to retract the curse, though, and his father had to learn to live with the mistake he made because of his short temper.

His mother tried her best to raise Ashtavakra a happy boy. However, going to school, or even going out of the house, was painful and difficult for him. He had no friends and no one said a kind word to him. He was teased by the other children. Although he grew up introverted and sad, he tried to remain optimistic. He worked hard and studied the Vedas and Vedanta. Having learned to handle a lot of pain, Ashtavakra grew up a wise person.

One day, he decided to go to King Janaka's court. He had heard of all the wise and learned men who were in the court and was eager to learn from them. It took him many days to travel to Janaka's court because his body moved very slowly. Finally, he arrived and entered the great hall where the court convened.

As soon as he entered, the entire court burst into laughter. As he looked around, Ashtavakra saw that the people assembled were openly pointing at him and laughing.

Ashtavakra looked at the assembly, dumbstruck. Soon, his body started to shake, seemingly with laughter. Seeing this, the entire court became puzzled and everyone grew quiet. King Janaka was the sole person in attendance who had not laughed. He spoke now.

'What makes you laugh?' he asked Ashtavakra.

'Oh, great king!' cried Ashtavakra. 'I had heard many legends about your court—the grandeur, the wise people, the righteousness. I undertook a long and arduous journey to attend it, only to find that those assembled here are mere shoemakers!'

'Shoemakers?' King Janaka was as puzzled as everyone else. 'You mean like cobblers?'

'Yes,' said Ashtavakra, wiping away his tears. 'A shoemaker only looks at the skin of a shoe and makes a judgement. These people also looked at my outer shell and laughed, never once thinking about how I would feel. You thought I was laughing when I was actually crying. There is sometimes a difference between what is and what appears to be true.'

Everyone assembled felt ashamed as it dawned on them that Ashtavakra was right. Whereas before they had been looking, pointing and laughing, now, they couldn't raise their eyes to meet anyone else's. They were embarrassed and contrite.

King Janaka was impressed. He continued conversing with Ashtavakra. The more he spoke to him, the more he realized that Ashtavakra was an uncommonly enlightened individual. In fact, King Janaka was so impressed by Ashtavakra that he became his disciple from then on.

SIGNIFICANCE AND SYMBOLISM

Throughout his life, Ashtavakra was laughed at and misunderstood because of his looks. Some people thought he was a scary miscreant while others thought he had a horrible disease. We all tend to be shoemakers—judging external appearances. Often, our first impressions are so strong that we have difficulty changing them.

This story emphasizes Ashtavakra's wisdom and intellect. But it is also important to note his perseverance. It was difficult for him to walk, yet, because he wanted to attend King Janaka's court, he undertook the journey. He had an aim, a goal in mind and was willing to work as hard as was required to achieve it. Similarly, the practice of yoga is fraught with difficulties. The Ashtanga system of yoga requires yogis to train their minds as much as their bodies, and this is a challenge.

However, like Ashtavakra, yogis should take no notice of discouragement and should make the effort required to stay on the path of yoga.

According to the Gita, the body is ephemeral, a mere shell, and the soul is eternal. The soul changes bodies the way we change clothes.

The body is cast off, like a snake sheds its skin. So it is important to look beyond the outer appearance of people and situations to see the light within. *Ashtavakrasana* is a reminder that yoga is not merely about the body, but also about the quest of the soul.

HOW TO

1. Sit on the floor with your legs extended.
2. Place your right leg on the arm right above the elbow. Place your right calf on top of the right shoulder.
3. Extend your left leg out between the arms.
4. Cross your legs at the ankles.
5. Bend your arms and lean forward, and lift your body up balancing on the arms
6. Repeat on the left side.

HELPFUL HINT

◈ This asana requires great hip flexibility as well as arm strength. Build up to it by first working on hip openers and a few basic arm balances.

BENEFITS

- Helps in aligning and balancing the body.
- Helps in cultivating arm and core strength.
- Increases the flexibility of the hip joint.

CONTRAINDICATIONS

This is an advanced asana and requires a combination of both flexibility and strength. Advanced and intermediate students can attempt this. Beginners should put in a few years of yoga practice before attempting this asana.

12

virasana

(hero's pose)

Many asanas are devoted to Hanuman, and with good reason. As the stories below show, Hanuman is the epitome of courage in the face of the highest danger, and commitment in the face of almost debilitating fear. The word *vir* means brave, strong and powerful. Hanuman repeatedly demonstrated these qualities and it earned him the moniker *mahavir*, the great hero. He is also called 'Vir Hanuman'.

THE GREATEST HERO OF THEM ALL

Hanuman met Lord Rama for the first time when Rama was in exile with Lakshmana and Sita. When his eyes fell on Lord Rama, he was overcome with devotion and immediately prostrated himself. As time went on and their relationship deepened, he felt a sense of responsibility towards the trio and devoted himself to their service.

One day, through clever deception, Ravana kidnapped Sita and took her to his kingdom of Lanka. Rama and Lakshmana immediately prepared for war and rallied their troops while Hanuman called his Vanar Sena, the monkey army. Everyone decided to join forces in the hunt for Sita.

Reaching Lanka would be a challenge. For many days and nights, they trekked through dense jungles and forests to go to the southernmost tip of India. This was the closest point to Lanka and they believed that from here, they could find their way. However, when they reached that point, they were confronted by a vast expanse of blue sea. They had no idea how to cross the sea. They also knew that Ravana's demon army awaited them on the other side. Having never fought them before, they didn't know what to expect. Everyone was worried and anxious.

Hanuman was a great devotee and had vowed to serve Rama, Lakshmana and Sita for the rest of his life. Being a great yogi, he was endowed with certain siddhis or powers. Using one such power, he took a deep breath and leapt across the large expanse of the unfamiliar ocean into Lanka. He had the demon army waiting for him on the other side, with only courage, valour, commitment, devotion and faith on his side. But that didn't discourage the brave Hanuman from coming to the rescue.

A GREAT FRIEND

When they found out that Sita had been kidnapped by Ravana and taken to Lanka, Rama and Lakshmana went after them without any delay. Hanuman followed them, bringing the Vanar Sena along with him. Together, they all went to Lanka. The battle that ensued was terrible, with skilled and brave warriors on both sides. Although Lakshmana was a talented warrior, he was severely injured during the battle and was rushed to the physician.

'The only thing that can save Lakshmana's life now is the herb Sanjeevani,' declared the physician sadly. 'If we don't obtain it before daybreak, then Lakshmana will be lost to us forever!' Everyone was speechless. Only Ravana rejoiced. He believed that if Lakshmana was indisposed, Rama would be easier to defeat, as Lakshmana was an important member of his force.

'I shall go find the herb,' declared Hanuman. He was a true friend and decided to take up the challenge. This proved to be no easy feat as Hanuman didn't know the location of the Sanjeevani herb. He knew it was in the Himalayas, but didn't know exactly where in the Himalayas. When Ravana found out that Hanuman was going to save the day once again, he shrewdly planted obstacles along his path that would hinder his progress. Hanuman, the great yogi, overcame every single one of these obstacles.

Seeing that Hanuman was winning and getting closer to the goal, Ravana had to think of another strategy. Since the physician had said that Lakshmana wouldn't survive until daybreak, Ravana went to Surya for help.

'O Surya,' he implored. 'Please come up early today and help me. I have great faith in your powers and have been a devotee for many years. I have done much penance and today, I look to you for help at a time of great difficulty. Please don't neglect me in my hour of need.'

But Hanuman was faster. He decided to expand in size to obliterate the sun. Now the onset of the day was delayed and Lakshmana could receive help in time.

Finally, Hanuman found an old lady who knew where the herb was located.

'Where can I find the Sanjeevani?' he asked her frantically.

The old lady tried her best to explain, but describing the location was proving to be difficult. Since they were running out of time, Hanuman decided to carry her on his shoulders and fly to the Himalayas. Once they got there, they saw numerous herbs growing everywhere on the mountain.

Unable to identify the Sanjeevani herb, and conscious that time was running out, Hanuman picked up the entire mountain and flew it back to Rama and Lakshmana in the nick of time. The physician was able to recognize and administer the herb.

With Lakshmana having returned from the jaws of death, Rama felt incredibly grateful to Hanuman and this cemented their bond further.

SIGNIFICANCE AND SYMBOLISM

There is much to learn from Hanuman. He was loyal to his friends, devoted to his causes, fixed on his purpose and reliable. Even today, seekers are encouraged to recite the *Hanuman Chalisa* to rid their minds of fear and to ward away dark forces.

Bravery isn't the absence of fear, it is the mastery of fear. Hanuman conquered his fear with faith to literally soar to new heights and perform noble deeds such as rescuing Sita. If we master our fears, we can also soar to great heights.

If Hanuman was the 'great hero', then why is he always depicted as sitting in a servile position in front of Rama? In some pictures, we see Hanuman with either one or both legs folded under him. While Hanuman knew that he had accomplished great feats, he was humble in front of his own hero, master and lord.

Regardless of how much success we achieve, we must always remain humble.

When practising *virasana*, we must try and find a balance between being aware of our accomplishments and accepting that there are many who are far greater and more accomplished than us. It is for us to humbly seek such individuals out and learn from them.

HOW TO

1. Kneel, keeping your feet hip-width apart.
2. Grab your calf muscles and rotate them outward.
3. Slowly lower yourself to the ground ensuring that the knees stay together.
4. Clasp your fingers and turn your hands outward so that your palms are facing the sky. Straighten your elbows.
5. Stretch your arms up and above your head, keeping them straight and the shoulders pushed down.

HELPFUL HINT

◎ In step three, many practitioners may not be able to lower themselves to the floor. In this case, place a bolster or a block under your hips. With regular practice, your knees will become more flexible and you will be able to lower yourself to the floor easily.

BENEFIT

◎ Maintains the flexibility of the lower body.
◎ Relieves back pain.
◎ Helps cure problems of the curvature of the back.
◎ Rests the legs and the lower body.

CONTRAINDICATIONS

Don't practice this asana if you're recovering from knee injuries.

13

marichyasana

(sage marichi's pose)

Marichi means ray of life. The story of Sage Marichi goes back to the creation of the universe.

THE POINT OF CREATION

As the creator of the universe, Lord Brahma shouldered a great responsibility. He understood the magnitude of the task entrusted to him. He knew that from planning to execution, everything must be done carefully.

He decided to start with creating Life. He wanted Life to have the ability to procreate and propagate itself. The first living beings he created were the Kumaras. However, the Kumaras were also endowed with free will and the ability to think. They considered Lord Brahma's request to procreate for the continuance of the universe and refused. They explained that they wanted to be celibate.

Brahma was in a fix. He realized he needed to create beings who understood the importance and necessity of the work he had undertaken. He needed living beings who were like-minded. He decided to create ten beings from his mind (*manasputra*) and nine from his body. The beings he created from his mind were also known as *prajapatis* and were the rulers of people. Marichi was one of the Prajapatis. All Prajapatis are the sons of Lord Brahma, and they are all incredibly powerful.

Marichi is also one of the saptarishis or the seven great rishis of the Hindu pantheon. The lineage he fathered at the behest of Brahma is illustrious and strong. His son was Sage Kashyap (also a saptarishi, but in a different era). His grandson is Surya—universally worshipped with the sun salutations. Manu, the first man, also regarded as the father of humanity, was Marichi's great-grandson. All the devas and asuras, even Ravana, are descendants of Marichi. Saptarishis change based on the yuga or the era. Hence, both Kashyap and his father Marichi were saptarishis.

As the universe started to take shape, Sage Marichi realized that he would have to choose between his worldly duties and the path of austerity and denunciation. Considering the enormity of the task Lord Brahma had undertaken and wanting to help him, he felt that he should prioritize his duties towards the creation of the universe.

A STRONG CURSE

Marichi had the power to cast spells and curses. At times, because of his short temper, his spells were unjust.

One day, Marichi came home very tired and requested his wife Dharmvrata to give him a foot massage. As Dharmvrata started the massage, Lord Brahma entered their house. Since he was a guest in their home, and he was Marichi's father, Dharmvrata knew she was supposed to look after his needs before the needs of anyone else in the household. So she stopped ministering to Marichi and enquired after Lord Brahma's well-being.

Perhaps because Marichi was very tired, he became livid at such a trifle. He was known for his wisdom, but he was also famous for the hasty decisions he made because of his short temper. He felt ignored by Dharmvrata and this incensed him.

'Dharmvrata!' Marichi thundered before he could control himself. 'You have offended not only your husband, but also a great saptarishi and prajapati. I shall curse you! Since you have shown such stony indifference to my needs, I condemn you to become a stone forever! You will be a rock, still and silent for all eternity!'

Dharmvrata was stunned and saddened in equal measure. She was also indignant because she hadn't done anything wrong. She decided to pray to Lord Vishnu to intervene. She was sure he could help release her from the unfair curse. After many years of prayers, Lord Vishnu was propitiated and manifested himself to her.

'I have noticed your long and hard *tapasya*,' Lord Vishnu said to Dharmvrata. 'What is your heart's desire? For such arduous penance, you deserve to be granted your wish. Tell me, what is it that you want?'

'O Lord Vishnu, you who sees everything,' she told him, 'my husband Marichi, Lord Brahma's son, has cursed me to be a stone for eternity! O Lord! Please end this curse and liberate me!'

'Alas!' Vishnu replied, 'Dharmvrata, your husband is so strong that it is impossible to undo his curse. But I can alleviate your suffering a little by modifying the curse. Although you will remain a stone, you will be considered holy. All the gods will desire you for your auspiciousness.'

And so Dharmvrata remains (even today) an auspicious, holy stone, cursed by her husband but desired by all the gods.

SIGNIFICANCE AND SYMBOLISM

In the kind of world we inhabit today, spiritual health has taken a backseat. One of the biggest challenges for us is to stay spiritual and grounded while living in a world that is becoming increasingly superficial and fast-paced. In the ideal world, people and circumstances would be perfect and there would be no wrong done to anyone. However, our world is less than perfect. Dharmvrata was punished for no fault of her own. She faced a curse for eternity due to Marichi's folly and was powerless to reverse it. But she persevered and tried all she could to alleviate her situation. Ultimately, she had to be content with a compromise.

The challenge in life is to make the most of situations. The key to doing that is to persevere through seemingly unyielding circumstances. If you do the right thing, you will reap the rewards of karma.

HOW TO

1.   Sit with your legs extended in front of you.
2.   Bending the right leg, place the right foot on the floor next to the left knee.
3.   Place your right hand on the floor behind you, twisting your torso to the right.
4.   Keep the left arm straight and elbow locked. Place the elbow on the outside of the right knee. Hold the left knee.
5.   Push with the left arm to deepen your twist. Exhale as you do so.
6.   Look over your right shoulder.
7.   Repeat on the left side.

HELPFUL HINT

◈   Practitioners have a tendency to curve the spine in this asana. This inhibits breathing and impedes the rotation of the torso. Keep your shoulders pushed back towards each other and away from the ears. Keep your chest open.

BENEFITS

◈   Enhances digestion.
◈   Helps flush toxins out of your system.
◈   Tones the abdominal muscles.

- Strengthens the abdominal organs.
- Relieves backache.

CONTRAINDICATIONS

In this asana, pressure is applied to the organs of digestion. So if you have diarrhoea, do not perform this. Also, don't perform it if you are pregnant.

dhanurasana
(page 88)

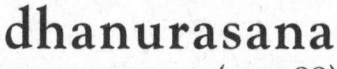

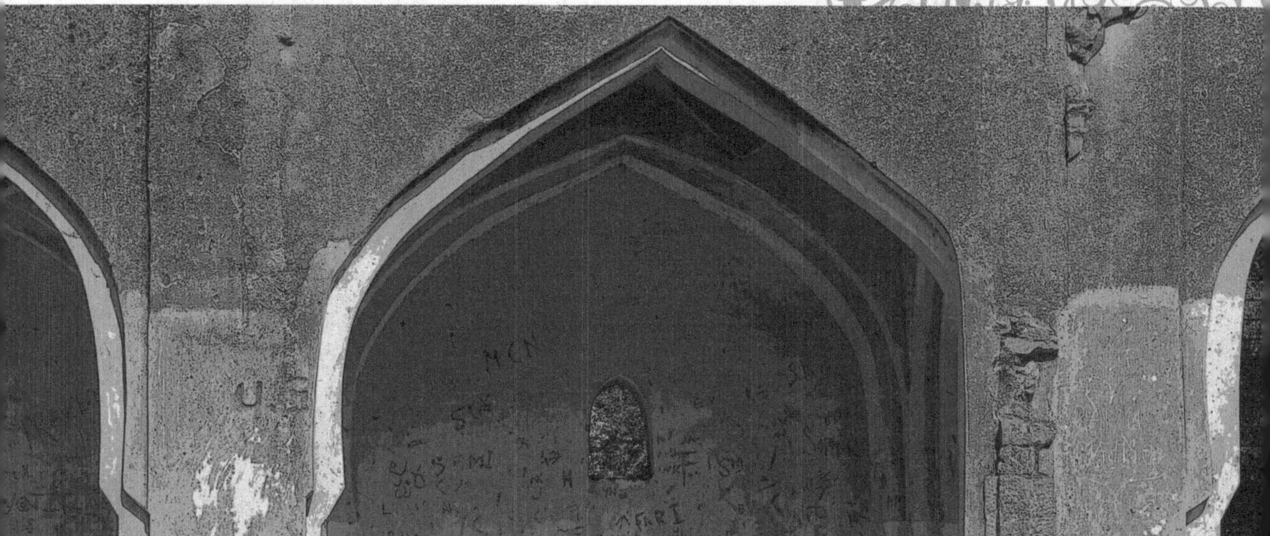

We must know when to push and when to pull ourselves back, so as not to get injured (in life and in our practice).

halasana
(page 93)

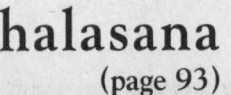

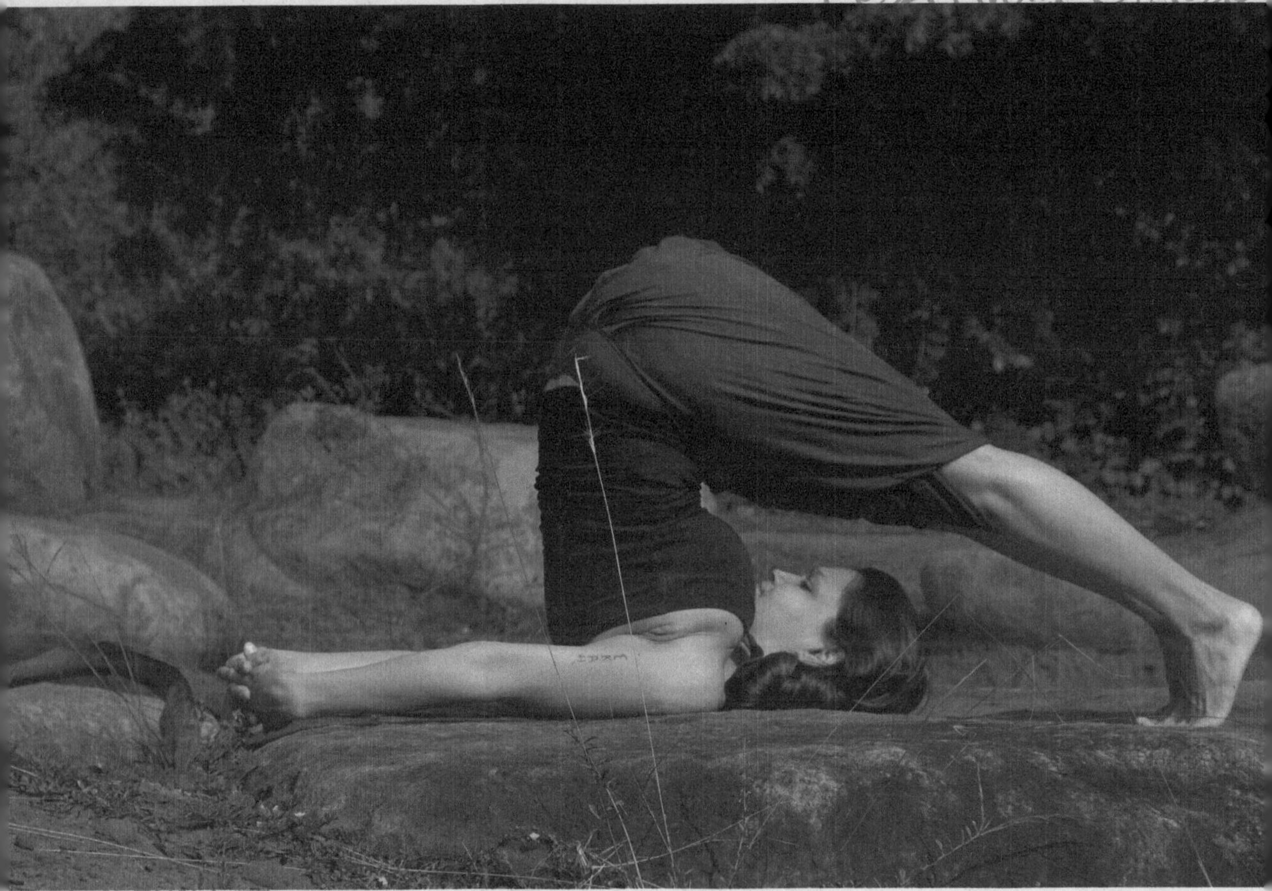

To learn new things, we must be open to changing or modifying the old, even unlearning the old and creating the new.

hanumanasana
(page 99)

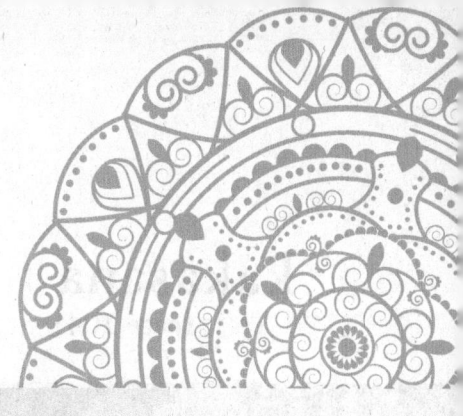

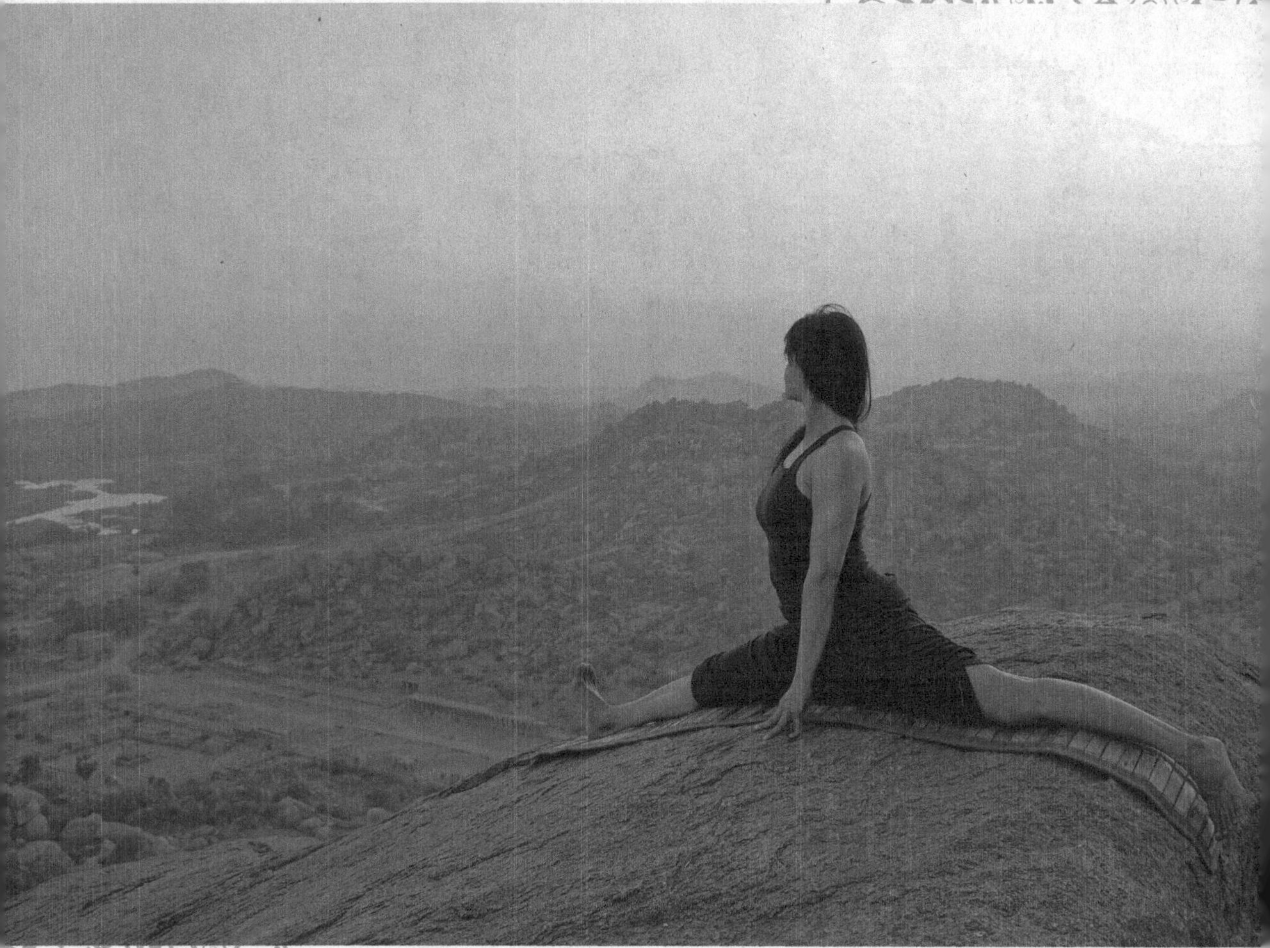

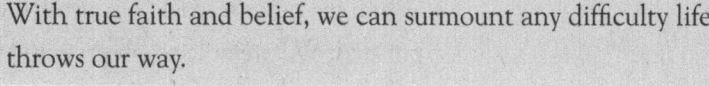

With true faith and belief, we can surmount any difficulty life throws our way.

kakasana

(page 104)

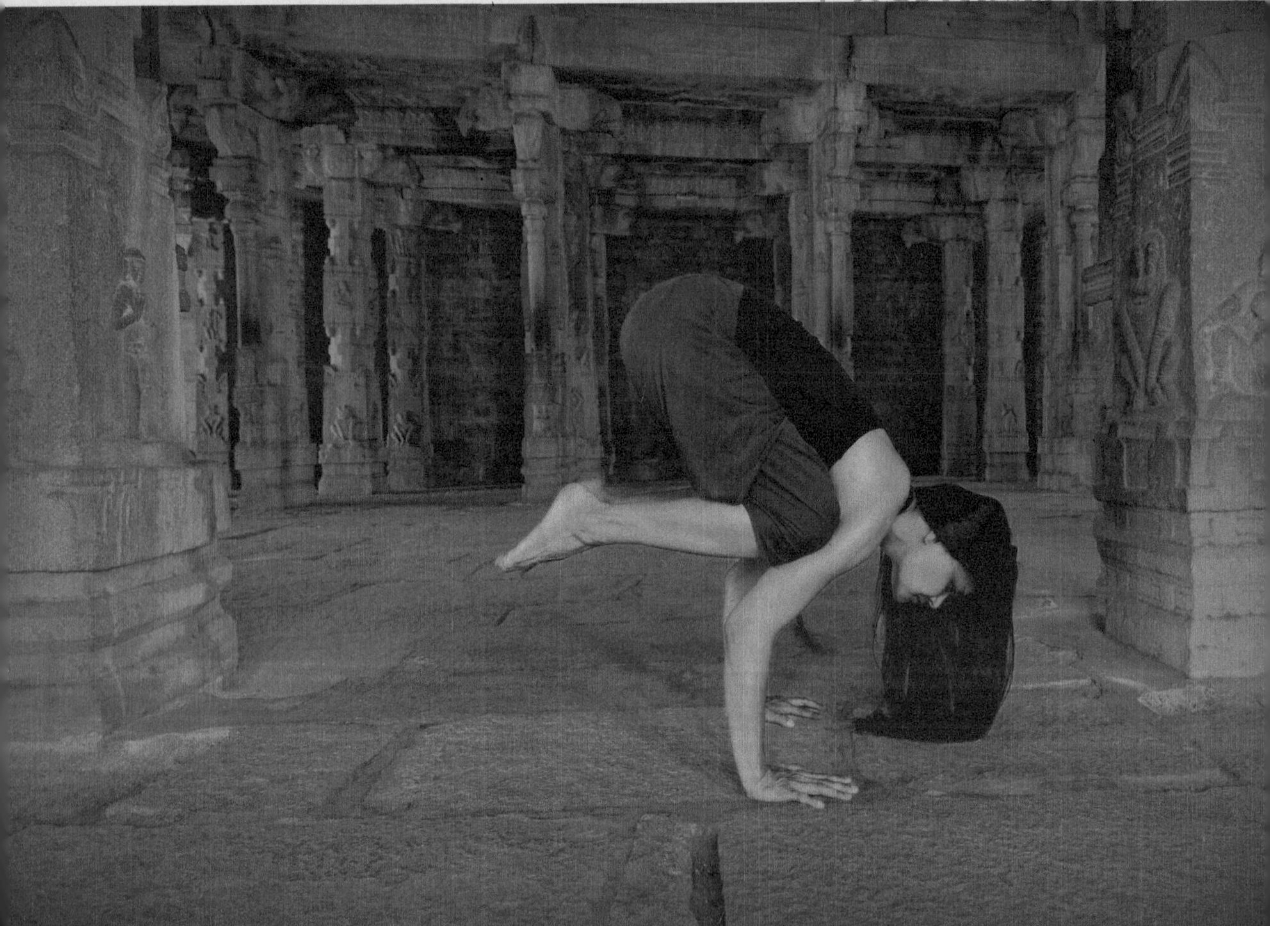

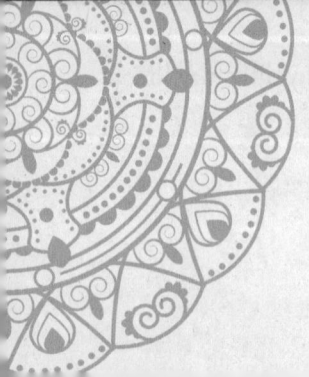

When we practise yoga, our intuition and perception are purified. We are able to observe and analyse more clearly. We learn to respond, rather than react, to situations.

kapotasana
(page 109)

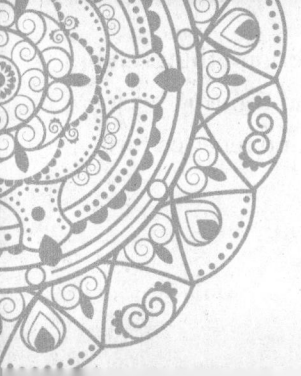

The purpose of yoga is to connect us to our innermost selves.

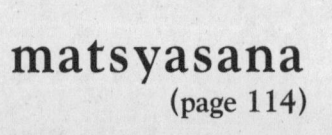

matsyasana
(page 114)

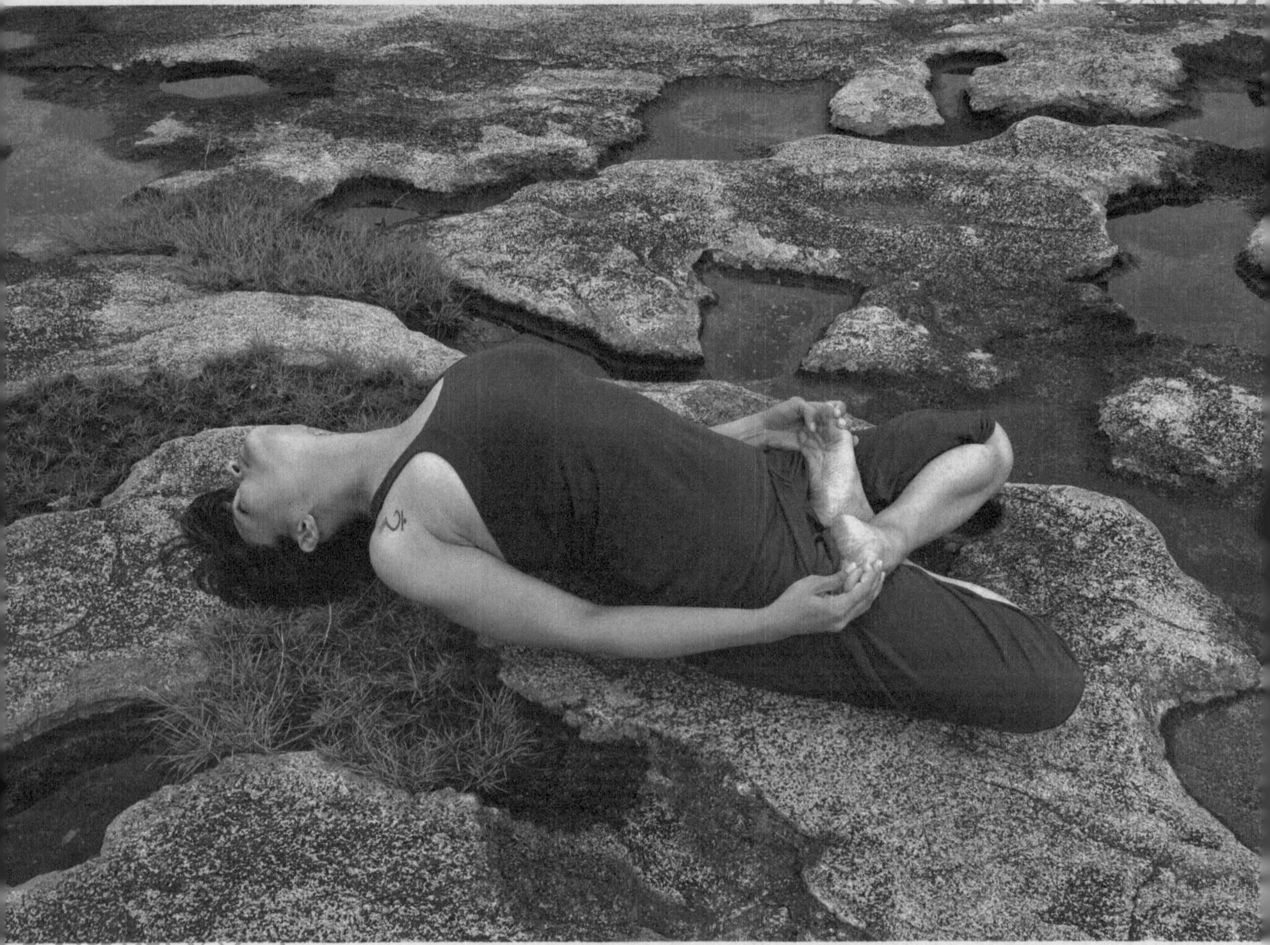

Every once in a while, we need to let go of emotions, things and even people that are not healthy, rewarding and constructive for us. This helps us move forward with freshness and renewed focus.

natrajasana

(page 119)

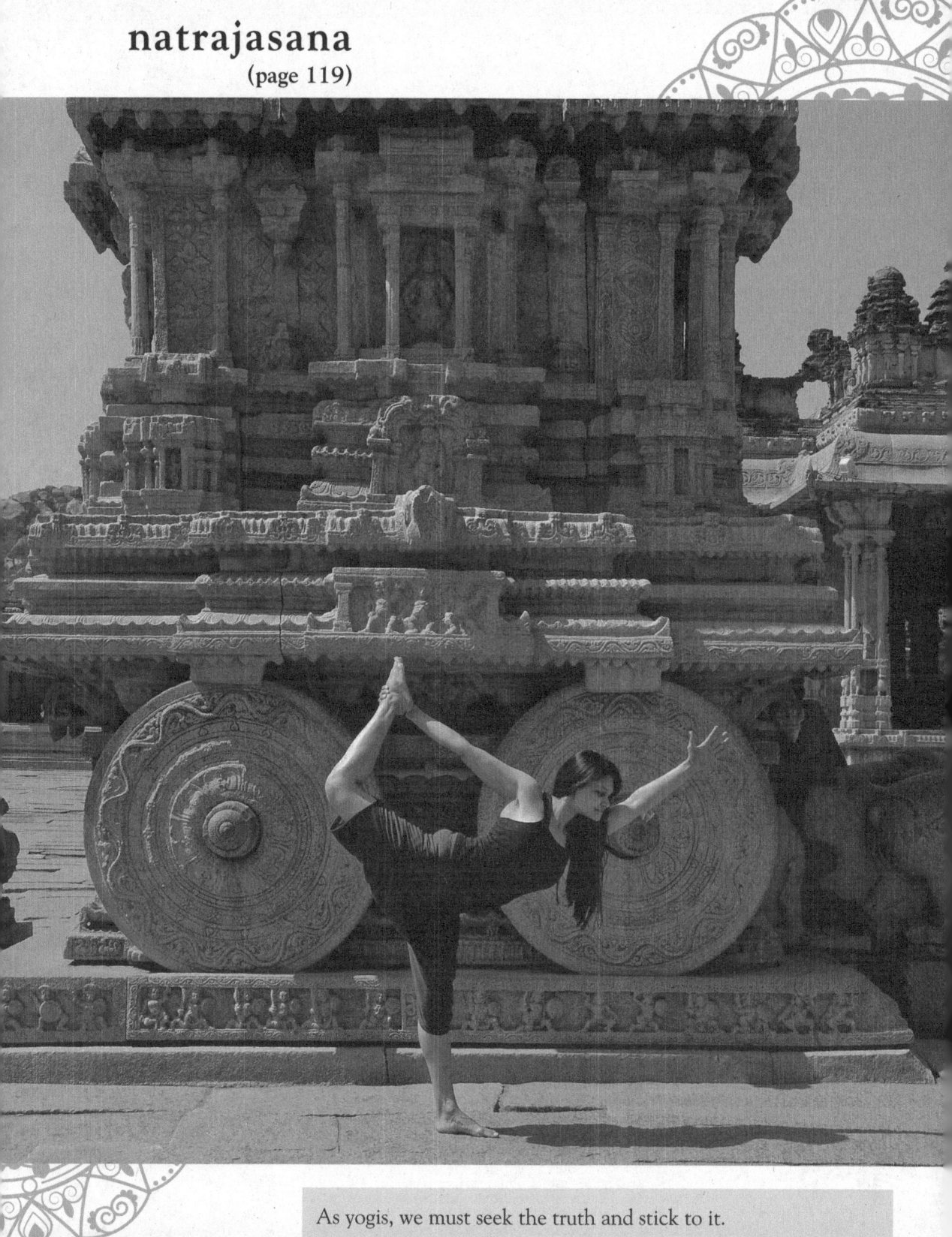

As yogis, we must seek the truth and stick to it.

sukhasana
(page 124)

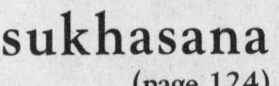

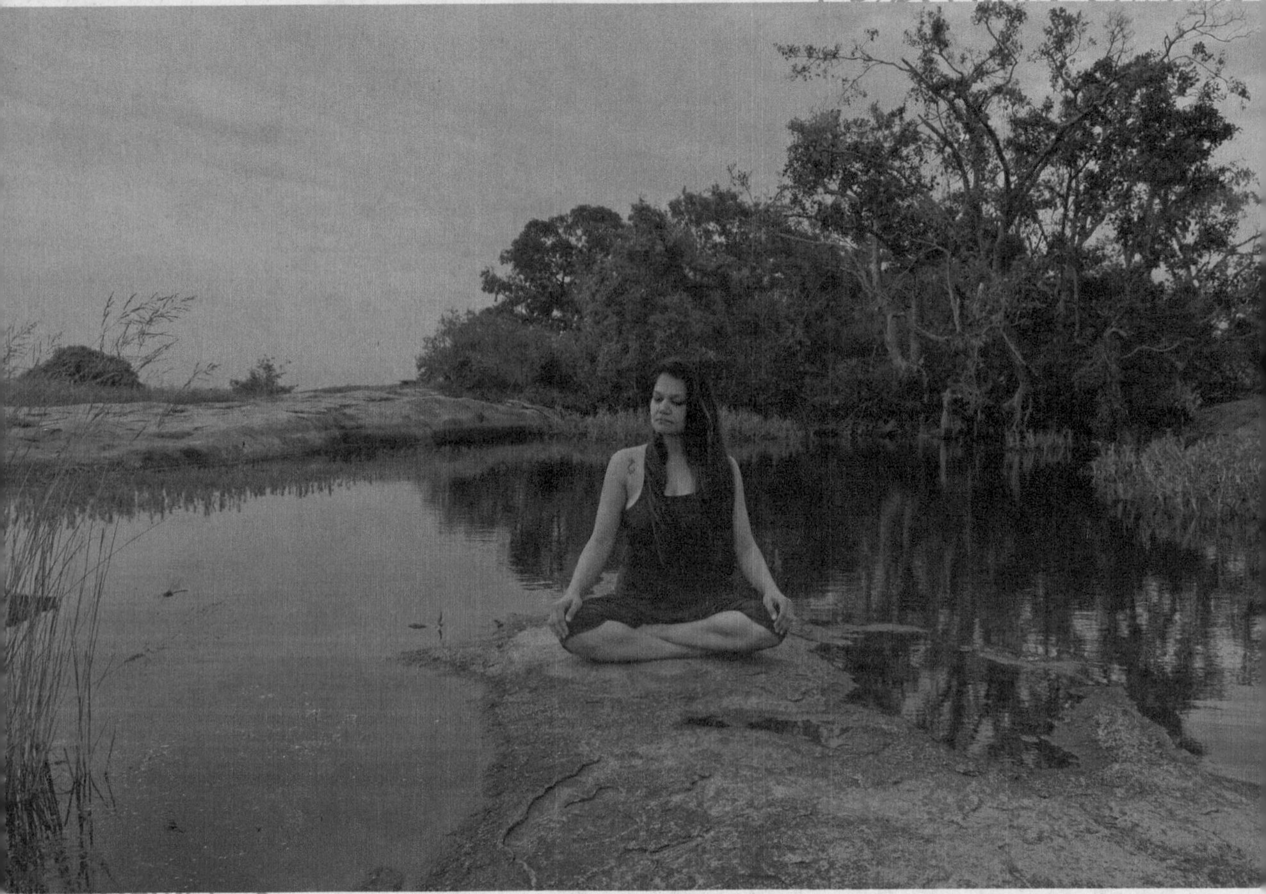

For progress, the practitioner must strike a balance between the comfort of practised moves and the uncertainty of new asanas. Discipline and correct practice alone will take us to the goal of yoga.

14

padmasana

(lotus pose)

The lotus is connected to all three deities of the Hindu trinity. Lord Vishnu has eyes like the lotus, Lord Brahma was born of the lotus and Lord Shiva always sits with his legs crossed in the padmasana.

The lotus represents beauty, grace and divinity. No wonder, then, that we can trace our origins to this exquisite flower.

CREATION

Before the creation of the universe, there existed only time. Time stretched and lengthened into nothingness; a vast emptiness.

Shakti, or energy, existed within time. This emptiness was meaningless and lacked beauty. It was a large canvas that could be used to express love. Shakti decided to use this canvas to create life and the universe. Shakti contained within her all the secrets of existence, including the secrets of the power of yoga. Using her yogic powers, she created a being who had the power to create and a being who had the power to destroy—Shiva and Vishnu. These two would balance each other. However, there had to be an energy that could sustain creation.

Life can't come out of nothingness. Life is a natural consequence of life itself. Shakti had a seed that contained the potential for life. There was also water, which could nurture and bring forth the life present within the seed. Shakti put the seed in the water and it germinated. Life manifested.

There was a lone lotus flower growing in Vishnu's navel. To nourish the seed further, Shakti put it inside the womb of this lotus. The flower bloomed and within it, the seed. Finally, Brahma, the creator, emerged from this seed.

Brahma went on to create the rest of the universe.

THE PADMA PURANA

The lotus is so significant that it is mentioned in the Rig Veda, the first text of Indian mythology. So important is the lotus that an entire Purana is named after it! This text is called the *Padma Purana*.

There are a total of eighteen Puranas and the *Padma Purana* is the second one. It is called the *Padma Purana* because it describes the important role the lotus played in the creation of the universe. Brahma, the creator, emerged from the lotus in Lord Vishnu's navel. The *Padma Purana* also details the spiritual practices that we should follow in order to achieve moksha. The Puranas are attributed to Ved Vyasa, who also wrote the Mahabharata.

The cornerstone of Hinduism is the large collection of texts related to its various traditions. These texts comprise stories of sages, rituals, beliefs, ethics, politics, art, etc. They have been relevant through the ages and provide insight and wisdom to seekers.

SIGNIFICANCE AND SYMBOLISM

A guru's feet are referred to as the 'lotus feet'. It is at the guru's feet that you will find enlightenment.

In yogic texts, there are innumerable references to the lotus flower. In the Gita, Lord Krishna exhorted people to strive to be like the lotus.

A lotus grows in muddy waters, but is never muddied. Similarly, we should be able to live in a world full of vices and temptations yet stay focused on the purpose of our lives.

There is much to learn from the lotus for yogis as well as non-practitioners. A lotus is rooted, like the mountains are rooted to the earth. But, unlike the mountains, the lotus started off as a small shoot in dirty water. It is unlikely for something so beautiful and graceful to emerge from muck, but the lotus flower, through sheer persistence, does so and blooms beautifully.

HOW TO

1. Sit with your legs stretched out in front of you.
2. Place the right foot on top of the left thigh, close to the left hip joint.
3. Do the same on the left leg, crossing it over the right leg.
4. Place your hands on your knees and keep your back straight.

HELPFUL HINTS

- If you're unable to place the foot close to your hip joint, then take a cushion and place it under your knee. The extra lift will help you get your leg in the right position.

- Sitting on a cushion will give you a slight forward tilt, which will help you raise and cross your legs easily.

BENEFITS

- Increases the flexibility and range of motion of the knees and ankles.
- Improves posture by straightening the back.
- The best pose for meditation.

CONTRAINDICATIONS

The padmasana is either very easy or a huge challenge for practitioners. Chances are you will experience pain when you try to position your legs in this asana. If this is due to an injury, then be gentle and patient. Start with small intervals and gradually increase the time you hold the pose.

15

bharadwajasana

(sage bharadwaj's pose)

Our desires and wants are a reflection of who we are. In the quest for 'more', we sometimes allow our desires to control us, instead of controlling our desires. Sometimes, we focus so intently on the object of our desire that we forget why we desired it in the first place.

Yoga helps us cultivate a sense of awareness. This awareness enables us to become cognisant of our *real* desires. As the experiences of Sage Bharadwaj show us, sometimes, we may not actually want what we think we do.

THE FRUITS OF LABOUR

Right from childhood, Bharadwaj had known that the only thing he liked to do was spend time studying and learning the Vedas. His parents encouraged his pursuits and as he grew up, his determination to master the Vedas strengthened. By the time he was in his teens, he knew he wanted to devote his entire life to the mastery of the Vedas.

Bharadwaj was a hard-working boy. Once he decided to master the Vedas, he stopped spending time with his friends. He sometimes forgot to eat and even to bathe. His parents tried, unsuccessfully, to interest him in family life, but Bharadwaj's only interest was to increase his knowledge of the Vedas every year. This gave him a wonderful sense of achievement.

Years passed. All his friends grew up, got married and had families of their own. Bharadwaj's parents grew old and eventually died. Yet, he continued his studies relentlessly.

Finally, when he lay on his deathbed, Lord Shiva appeared to him. He was pleased with the hard work Bharadwaj had done. When Bharadwaj saw Lord Shiva, he was incredulous. When he realized that this wasn't a dream, he became overjoyed. He had one last wish and he hoped Lord Shiva would grant it.

'O Lord Shiva, you have seen how much penance I have done my entire life,' he said. 'I have eschewed the luxuries of family life and other worldly comforts. I have devoted everything I have to the pursuit of knowledge. I have achieved a high degree of mastery in the study of the Vedas. I have only one more wish. Please, O Great One, grant me my last and final wish.'

'What is it that you want?' asked Lord Shiva.

'I wish to be liberated from the shackles of birth and rebirth and attain moksha. I have worked night and day to learn all there is to know about the Vedas. I have mastered all the stories and the lessons too. There is not a single person who knows more about the Vedas than I do. I have achieved more than anyone can achieve in a lifetime and I want to now enjoy moksha.'

'Bharadwaj,' said Lord Shiva, 'It is true that in your lifetime, you have studied more than anyone else and you deserve to be rewarded for it. But the reward can't be moksha. For true liberation, you must share your knowledge with other seekers. That is the true purpose of the acquisition of knowledge. Knowledge in and of itself is of no use unless it can uplift others and enlighten them.'

Bharadwaj was crestfallen.

'Don't despair, Bharadwaj,' said Lord Shiva. 'You have achieved great success in your lifetime. But also remember, our Vedas are vast, and the amount you have learnt is a handful of dirt compared to the mountain of knowledge that exists!'

Bharadwaj was now severely disappointed.

'O Shiva,' he said, 'I feel my entire life has been useless and all my work has come to nought.'

Seeing his plight, Lord Shiva felt compassion. 'Okay, Bharadwaj, I will give you one more chance to attain moksha. In your next life, alongside the pursuit of knowledge, help others uplift themselves by sharing your knowledge.'

Bharadwaj fell to Lord Shiva's feet, feeling very grateful, happy and relieved.

And so it was that in his next life, Bharadwaj spent his time teaching. He helped students understand the Vedas as he understood them. He encouraged his students when they felt demotivated, taught them how to think independently and was always available to answer their questions. He spent as much time sharing his knowledge as he did assimilating it. Soon, word of his accomplishments spread far and wide and his fame grew.

As the years passed, he continued teaching with the same zeal and enthusiasm. He taught until he was frail and weak and could no longer bear the physical strain of teaching. When he was on his deathbed, students came from all over the world to pay homage to him. Bharadwaj felt happy, fulfilled and satisfied.

Finally, Lord Shiva appeared again.

'I am proud of you, Bharadwaj,' he said, smiling. 'You have not only learned your lesson, but have also gained profound and unparalleled wisdom in the process. You are a legendary teacher who has made an impact on the lives of your students by imparting valuable lessons to them. Now you are truly ready for mukti, and I shall grant it to you!'

However, Bharadwaj had other plans. A lifetime of teaching and sharing his knowledge had given him insight into what he truly desired. He had enjoyed himself so much that he wanted to continue spending several more lifetimes teaching and enlightening students.

'You were right, O Wise One,' he said to Lord Shiva. 'Knowledge is of no value unless it is shared and used to uplift others. I see real merit and usefulness in teaching.

Rather than withdrawing from the cycle of birth and death, I would like to spend all eternity teaching and sharing my knowledge.'

Lord Shiva was proud of him and blessed him for his noble journey.

SIGNIFICANCE AND SYMBOLISM

As explained earlier, the word 'yoga' comes from the root 'yuj', which means to 'yoke' or to 'unite'.

The practice of yoga teaches us to slow down and observe ourselves. It teaches us to recognize and align ourselves with what we truly want. Asana is only one of the eight limbs of the Ashtanga system of yoga, and it focuses on the physical well-being of the practitioner. The remaining limbs focus on the holistic development of a human being.

Sometimes, our focus shifts from the deeper purpose of yoga to rest only on the physical practice of asana. We forget why we practise yoga and become obsessed with external pursuits such as perfection in asanas. Similarly, Bharadwaj never stopped to consider the greater purpose of accumulating knowledge. Shiva was enlightened and knew the best way to guide Bharadwaj towards the righteous path. And once Bharadwaj took that path, he found his true calling. True emancipation for him lay in sharing his knowledge with others to help them elevate themselves. He was willing to give up moksha to continue the work he loved doing and serve mankind.

When he was thinking of moksha, Sage Bharadwaj was only thinking of himself. When he decided to use his skills for the greater common good, he was thinking of society. Compassion and kindness are the basic maxims for yogis, and when Bharadwaj was able to comprehend these, he became a true yogi and eligible to receive the fruits of enlightenment.

Yoga is a mysterious journey and reveals its secrets over time. The practitioner must remain sincere and honest to the practice. Only with these elements will the power of yoga work for us. Like Bharadwaj, we may also find a sense of purpose in the quest for alignment in our lives. We must work on aligning our actions with our thoughts.

Once our thoughts are aligned, we must try to align our worlds. When there is alignment, there is a sense of balance. And that is the true purpose of yoga.

HOW TO

1. Sit on the floor with your legs extended.
2. Bend your right leg in marichyasana (see Chapter 13).
3. Fold it under you in half-virasana (see Chapter 12).
4. Fold the left leg in half-padmasana (see Chapter 14).
5. Place the right hand on the left knee and twist your torso to the right.
6. Reach back and hold the left foot with the left hand.
7. Repeat on the other side.

HELPFUL HINT

◎ If you are unable to reach the left foot, place your hand on the floor behind you.

BENEFITS

◎ Helps in relieving sciatica pain.
◎ Strengthens and stretches the back and abdominal muscles.
◎ Improves posture and breathing.

◉ Helps in maintaining and increasing the flexibility of the joints of the
   lower body.

CONTRAINDICATIONS

The *bharadwajasana* is a deep spinal twist and engages the abdominal muscles and the sides. This asana also engages your abdominal organs and the ribcage. It is important for you to have healthy knees, shoulders and hips to perform this asana. Don't perform this asana if you are recovering from injuries in the joints of the lower body or the shoulders, or recuperating from surgery on the abdominal organs.

16

bhujangasana

(serpent pose)

Snakes are usually feared and dreaded, but they hold a special place in Hindu mythology. Although considered inauspicious by many, snakes have repeatedly helped and cooperated with the devas and asuras. Because of their significant role in mythology, snakes also find mention in yoga lore.

SNAKES AND BELTS

Readers will remember Lord Ganesh and his run-in with a snake on his way home from a feast. At that time, it was a snake that caused him to lose all the sumptuous food he had eaten, but the same snake enabled him to gather up the food again and continue on his merry way. The story goes that one day, Lord Ganesh was invited to a huge feast. He loved to eat and there was a lot of delicious food and drink there. He enjoyed himself to the hilt, and drank and ate like there was no tomorrow. In fact, he overate. On his way home, he was perched on his ride, Krauncha the mouse, when a snake slithered across their path, startling them both. Krauncha's rhythmic gait was disrupted and Ganesh toppled over. As he landed heavily on the floor, his belly burst open and all the food he had consumed fell out. Ganesh was dismayed because he had enjoyed the food and wanted all of it in his stomach! He picked up every single item of food and put it back in his stomach. Then he reached for the snake that had caused the fall and tied it around his waist to secure the food in his belly.

Happy and satisfied, he continued on his way home.

SNAKE TO THE RESCUE

Many years ago, Lord Indra offended Durvasa by accidentally insulting the gift of a garland of flowers that Durvasa had given him. Furious, Durvasa cursed him, rendering the devas powerless. Soon, they started losing all their battles to the asuras. It was imperative that balance be restored, and so the devas made a pact with the asuras. They would share the nectar of immortality or amrit, which lay under the ocean, with the asuras, but on one condition. They would have to help them churn the ocean to draw the amrit out. The asuras agreed and thence began the great Samudra Manthan, the churning of the ocean.

Eventually, the devas realized that they would need more help for the task. Mount Mandara was recruited and Vasuki, the powerful snake, was asked to help by serving as the rope.

The devas had a devious plan. They held Vasuki's tail and told the asuras to hold his head. Vasuki got progressively dizzier as the churning continued, until, finally, hot fumes started issuing from his mouth. The fumes increased and before they realized what was happening, the asuras melted away! In some versions of the story, the poison that came out of Vasuki's mouth next was the halahala, and even more deadly. It had the capacity to destroy the world. Thankfully, Lord Shiva saw this in the nick of time and took the poison into his mouth, intending to swallow it. But Parvati grabbed and squeezed his neck hard, so the poison didn't descend into his belly and kill him. The poison turned Lord Shiva's throat blue, earning him the moniker Neelkanth.

THE SNAKE WHO BECAME A SAGE

Lord Vishnu was once reclining on Adishesha (Lord of the Serpents), and watching Lord Shiva dance. His dance was so enchanting that Lord Vishnu was completely absorbed. His body began to sway languidly to the rhythm of the dance movements. As he relaxed and allowed the movements to engulf his body, he started becoming heavier. Adishesha found it increasingly difficult to support his weight and was about to collapse. Just at that moment, Lord Shiva's dance ended and Vishnu's body became light again.

Puzzled by this, Adishesha asked Lord Vishnu the reason.

'The grace, beauty, majesty and grandeur of Shiva's dance is so mesmerizing that anyone who watches it is always hypnotized,' explained Vishnu. 'Their bodies start to relax and sway automatically.' Impressed, Adishesha decided he wanted to learn to dance like Shiva.

'I too would like to gain such mastery over the art of dance, my Lord,' said Adishesha. 'Please tell me how I can learn.'

Lord Vishnu thought deeply about this. He meditated for a long time in search of the answer. Such a noble desire must be fulfilled. Finally, one day, he found the answer.

'Adishesha, you are destined to write a commentary on grammar. And Lord Shiva himself will ask you to do so! You can then devote yourself to the perfection of the art of dance.'

Hearing this, Adishesha's joy knew no bounds. He at once began to meditate to find out how he would be manifested on Earth.

A vision of the yogini Gonika came to him. Gonika was praying for a worthy son to whom she could impart her knowledge and wisdom. He realized that she would be the perfect mother to him. She had also been praying for many years, and as a last resort, had prayed to Surya to fulfil her desires. Taking a handful of water in her hands, she closed her eyes and meditated upon the sun. When she was about to offer the water, she opened her eyes and saw a tiny snake in her hands, which slowly morphed into a human being. This tiny human prostrated himself in front of Gonika and asked her to accept him as her son. She did and called him 'Patanjali' (*pata* meaning falling or fallen, and *anjali*, oblation or hands folded in prayer).

SIGNIFICANCE AND SYMBOLISM

Snakes are a great contradiction.

On one hand, they inspire fear and symbolize death. On the other, they have helped the gods time and time again. Mere mortals are terrified of snakes, but not the gods. They are powerful, and have absolute control over and can calmly commune with snakes.

The practice of yoga teaches us to be disciplined and to master our fears.

Snakes are a metaphor for our fears and negative emotions. We should try and accept our fears and resolve our negative emotions. This is important because our fears can sometimes be debilitating and can discourage us from reaching for our goals.

The shedding of the snake's skin is powerfully symbolic. It signifies resurrection, renewal and rebirth.

Life and situations require us to renew, rethink and reinvent ourselves. Growth can only happen if we shed the old and insignificant and walk towards the new. We must endeavour not to dwell on the past, or on inconsequential things, and always try to look the current situation straight in the face. We must jettison all that does not serve us and keep only that which is valuable and conducive to our spiritual development.

HOW TO

1. Lie on your stomach and place your hands on either side of your chest.
2. As you inhale, push your hands into the floor and raise your torso. Engage your back muscles to lift and lengthen the torso.
3. Expand your chest by rotating your shoulders back.

HELPFUL HINT

- Many practitioners have a tendency to put all their weight on their hands. This puts too much stress on the wrists and weakens them. To correct this tendency and improve this asana, visualize a snake. A snake has no arms and has to rely on its muscles to lift and open its hood. Use your arms minimally when lifting the torso.

BENEFITS

- Stretches and tones the abdominal muscles and organs.
- Strengthens the back muscles.
- Conditions the spine and keeps it healthy.

CONTRAINDICATIONS

This asana engages the abdomen. Stretching tender muscles can retard the healing process, so if you are recovering from stomach ulcers, or from an abdominal surgery, avoid this asana. Never practise this during pregnancy.

17

dhanurasana

(bow pose)

Yoga is a *sadhaka*'s (student's) journey to peace, self-realization and, finally, nirvana. It is ironic, then, that there is an asana named after a weapon, which is a tool for destruction. Anything that can be misused can also be used. A weapon can be used to fight a war or to maintain peace. And as we see in the following stories, bows have meant more than just weapons of war.

A BOW EACH

In some books of the Hindu scriptures, Lord Vishwakarma is described as being responsible for the creation of the universe. He was known as the 'Principal Architect of the Universe', the very personification of creation. As he was planning and creating the universe, he realized that the entity he was creating was complex and unpredictable. For the universe to endure, there had to be ways to ensure its continuation, or it would perish. He realized that if he didn't create a system of checks and balances, the universe that he had so lovingly created might self-destruct one day. With this foresight, he understood that to maintain peace in the universe, war was necessary. And hence, there was a need of powerful instruments that could aid righteous warriors in waging important wars.

He crafted two invincible bows. Those who possessed them would have unmatched power. So powerful were these bows, in fact, that they had to be returned to their cases after use, for their power could destroy everything around them if left unsupervised. He also knew that he would have to be supremely careful about whom he gave them to. He decided that he would give one to Lord Shiva and one to Lord Vishnu. Lord Shiva's bow came to be called Pinaka and Vishnu's, the Sharanga. Time and time again, these bows played crucial roles in enabling righteousness to prevail.

WINNING HEARTS

Draupadi was the most beautiful princess in the kingdom and all the princes wanted to marry her. Finally, she came of age, and the time came for her to wed. King Drupada, her father, arranged for a *swayamvar*, as was the custom in those days. Drupada was a respected king. He understood that everyone had been waiting for Draupadi's swayamvar. He wanted only the noblest husband for his daughter. The only way to ensure that he got the best was to test the princes.

He devised a difficult challenge.

The challenge was that the prospective suitor had to take aim and shoot an arrow through the eye of a revolving fish while looking at the reflection of the fish in water. Drupada had a special contraption (*yantra*) in the shape of a fish constructed specially for the swayamvar. He called it Matsyayantra. The Matsyayantra would move in a circle and would be reflected in the water in a vessel on the ground below it. Eligible suitors had to look at the reflection and shoot the Matsyayantra in the eye as it moved!

The bow to be used for this great contest was Pinaka, Lord Shiva's bow.

One by one, the valiant princes tried their luck, but no one was able to even lift the bow, much less string it to take aim! Finally, it was Arjuna's turn. He easily picked up the bow and took perfect aim. And with that, he won the hand and the heart of a legendary beauty.

In this way, Pinaka played a significant role in one of the most celebrated episodes in the Mahabharata.

A FINE WARRIOR

Arjuna was an excellent warrior. He spent many years perfecting the usage of the bow. His guru was Dronacharya, who was tasked with teaching marksmanship and war games to Arjuna and his brothers. Arjuna far outstripped his brothers in all skills and his fame grew far and wide.

Dronacharya was an exacting teacher and would frequently test his pupils. One day, he decided to give Arjuna and his brothers one such test. He pointed to a sparrow sitting on a tree and asked the brothers to take aim at the eye of the bird.

Dronacharya: What do you see?

Yudhishthira: I see everything—the bird, the branch, the tree, even the clouds and the grass.

Nakula: I see everything too. Even the flowers and the other trees.

Bheema: I see everything too, even the other branches of the tree and the clouds as well.

Arjuna: I see only black—the blackness of the pupil of the sparrow's eye.

This keen eye and attention to detail is what distinguished Arjuna as a fine marksman.

SIGNIFICANCE AND SYMBOLISM

In the *dhanurasana*, we pull our hands back to resemble a bow. The '*dhanur*' or bow is a symbol of strength. We must channelize the strength and power of this symbol. The yogi's mind and body should be strong and indestructible. To take aim and hit the bullseye, we must use our bows, our bodies and our minds to stay focused on and unwavering from the righteous path.

This pose is also about balance. With a real bow, if you pull the string too hard, you may end up breaking it. And if you don't pull the string enough, you won't be able to launch the arrow. Arjuna was a great warrior because he instinctively understood the fine balance needed to hit the target.

Similarly, we must know when to push and when to pull ourselves back, so as not to get injured (in life and in our practice).

There are many kinds of bows in literature. We know from popular lore that Cupid's and Kamadeva's bows have caused many problems when not used wisely. In mythology, however, warriors have used bows responsibly. The bow of a saw and the bow of a violin are similar, but they create different things.

As humans, we need to recognize what we are aiming for. And like Arjuna, we need to stay focused on the target and not let our minds or eyes waver from that target.

We must ensure that our goals are noble and behave keeping good karma and deeds in mind.

HOW TO

1. Lie on your stomach.
2. Bend your right leg and reach back to hold the right ankle with the right hand.
3. Do the same with your left leg, holding the ankle with the left hand.
4. Now lift your thighs up off of the floor and leverage the strength in your legs to pull your torso up.
5. Keep your neck long and relax your shoulders.

HELPFUL HINT

- Practitioners have a tendency to splay the knees. Keep your knees and thighs not more than hip width apart.

BENEFITS

- Stimulates digestive organs.
- Tones and strengthens the abdominal muscles and spine.
- Massages and stimulates the thyroid gland.
- Stretches the arms, shoulder blades and chest.

CONTRAINDICTIONS

The dhanurasana requires a lot of weight to be borne by the abdomen, so it is advisable not to practice if you have stomach ulcers or have had a recent abdominal surgery.

18

halasana

(plough pose)

The practice of yoga is as much, if not more, about cultivating the mind as the body. We can shape and form our mind by ploughing deep into its recesses. A healthy mind gives rise to healthy thoughts. Healthy thoughts lead to a healthy life. As the stories below show, our thoughts actually do shape our world.

DISCOVERY OF A DAUGHTER

King Janaka was a compassionate and just ruler. He cared deeply about his kingdom and was revered by all his subjects.

However, a great sadness afflicted King Janaka and his wife Sunayna. They were childless and desperately yearned to have a child. For many years, they had tried to propitiate the gods by doing arduous penance, but all in vain.

They grew increasingly distraught. Seeing their king and queen unhappy, the subjects also felt sad. The king's state of mind affected the administration of his kingdom. Soon, the crops also dried up. The kingdom was slowly deteriorating.

King Janaka was in a fix. There was a severe drought across the kingdom. He realized that if he didn't do something soon, his kingdom may perish forever. Feeling guilty about having avoided his duty, he threw himself into controlling the damage he felt was his doing.

However, try as he might, he was unable to fix things. King Janaka became even more depressed. Not only was his kingdom in shambles, but he remained childless. He decided to do the biggest penance of all. He would plough the barren fields of his kingdom himself until the gods were satisfied and sent rain to revive the parched land.

Little did he know that a surprise awaited him as he toiled under the hot and harsh sun.

Busy and distracted as he was by his thoughts, Janaka almost missed the cries of a baby coming from the earth he was ploughing. The cries got louder until they finally penetrated Janaka's thoughts. Upon investigation, he discovered the most beautiful baby girl in one of the grooves on the earth. His joy knew no bounds. He was mesmerized by the little hands and feet. He held the baby girl to his chest and tried to calm her down. He comforted her and wiped away her tears. As he held the baby lovingly in his arms, King Janaka decided to adopt her. He took her home to an overjoyed Sunayna and named her Janaki.

She also came to be known as Sita.

THE PREFERRED WEAPON

Lord Krishna's son Samba had always been naughty. As he grew up, he became more reckless and difficult to control. Although good at heart, he frequently let his heart control his actions. Balrama, Krishna's brother, knew his nephew's weaknesses, but loved him anyway. He was a devoted uncle who doted on his nephews.

Samba would go on to test his family's patience severely.

Being reckless and high-strung, he fell in love with Lakshmana, Duryodhan's daughter. Lakshmana was a nice girl who was also beautiful and intelligent. Samba wanted to marry her. He waited patiently, if a little restlessly, for her to come of age.

When it was finally time for her to get married, her father arranged for her to have a swayamvar, as was the custom at the time. Being a loving and responsible father, Duryodhan planned the swayamvar with great care. He was proud of his daughter's compassionate nature and great beauty, and hopeful of a deserving husband for her. On the day of the swayamvar, all the princes from the neighbouring kingdoms came to win Lakshmana's hand in marriage.

Before the swayamvar could begin, Samba kidnapped Lakshmana. All hell broke loose.

Duryodhan sent his brothers with his best warriors to rescue his daughter. By kidnapping Lakshmana from right under his nose, Samba had publicly insulted him. This was an affront to him, his dignity, his kingdom and all his guests! He wanted revenge.

As the search for Samba and Lakshmana continued, Duryodhan was sick with worry for his daughter. He had heard of Samba and his infamous reputation and was afraid for his daughter. When the search party finally found them, Samba put up a good fight. But Duryodhan's men were experienced warriors and easily overpowered him. They captured him and took him prisoner.

When he heard this, Krishna was livid. He saw this as an insult to their entire dynasty. Krishna wanted to declare war on Duryodhan's kingdom, but Balrama cautioned him.

'Let's try and reason it out with Duryodhan,' Balrama said. 'Any father would react like this if his daughter had been kidnapped. Now that he has his daughter back, we can calmly convince him to let Samba go.'

Balrama took a small party and requested an audience with Duryodhan.

'I understand your anger, Duryodhan,' said Balrama. 'But what is done is done. As much as I would like to change what has happened, I can't. But we can discuss the best course of action now and ensure it is agreeable to everyone.'

'What course could possibly be agreeable to all of us?' thundered Duryodhan. 'My daughter was disgraced at her own swayamvar. I was shamed in front of the princes from the neighbouring kingdoms. My guests were dishonoured and I sat watching helplessly. My daughter will have to live with this ignominy for the rest of her life.'

'We will convince Samba to free Lakshmana,' offered Balrama. 'Then you can continue with the swayamvar!'

'Don't talk like you're ignorant of the rules,' scoffed Duryodhan. 'You know that a woman who is abducted becomes the property of her abductor and will never have a swayamvar.'

Balrama thought hard about the problem. 'Samba abducted Lakshmana because he wishes to marry her, so why don't we get them married?'

'We know they like each other,' Balrama continued. 'Then why not let them be wedded? This will solve everyone's problem.'

Although Duryodhan heard the wisdom in his words, his ego was unwilling to concede to the logic. The more Balrama reasoned, the more intractable Duryodhan became. Finally, he rudely dismissed Balrama and his party from the kingdom. Now Balrama got angry. Seizing his plough, he spoke to the gathered court. 'Either we reach a compromise right now, or I harm your city!' Duryodhan was deaf to all entreaties, threats and warnings.

Balrama and his party left. When they exited the precincts of the kingdom of Hastinapur, he grabbed his plough and plunged it deep into the ramparts of the city. He pulled the plough away, and the ramparts along with it. Without its bearings, the city of Hastinapur started to tilt into the Ganges.

As he felt the ground tilting under him, Duryodhan realized that they must call for a truce or his kingdom would perish forever.

And even today, if you look at the city of Hastinapur, you will notice that it is tilted slightly to the side, towards the Ganges.

SIGNIFICANCE AND SYMBOLISM

The plough is an ambivalent symbol. It can be a weapon or a useful tool. When Balarama decided to use his plough, he forced it into the earth, breaking it open to commit an act of violence. King Janaka also used the plough in the same manner, but he used it to sow the land to create nourishment and growth.

The circumstances and events in our lives are the ploughs. It is up to us to use them to either generate growth or to escalate decay.

The same event can be greeted with sadness by some and jubilation by others.

When it comes to the daily physical practice of yoga, we have to be willing to push through the pain and discomfort. Progress lies beyond the comfort zone.

Just like the earth needs to be ploughed periodically to remain fertile, our minds and bodies must be constantly challenged to remain open, receptive and flexible.

Soil should be neither too hard nor too soft to be fertile. Similarly, people shouldn't be too hard nor too soft.

To learn new things, we must be open to changing or modifying the old, even unlearning the old and creating the new.

HOW TO

1. Lie on your back.
2. Bend your legs and bring your knees close to your chest.
3. Engage your abdominal muscles and lift your buttocks up. Support your back with your hands.
4. Continue to lift your buttocks until your spine is perpendicular to the floor.
5. Slowly extend your legs out over your head and touch the toes to the floor.

HELPFUL HINT

- If you are unable to touch the floor with your toes, prop your feet up on a stool or chair.

BENEFITS

- Relaxes the mind and increases energy.
- Relaxes the eyes and brain.
- Increases blood circulation.
- Provides relief from hypertension.
- Improves digestion.
- Stretches and relaxes the spine.
- Reduces insomnia, anxiety, migraines.
- Provides a great stretch for the shoulders and neck.

CONTRAINDICATIONS

The *halasana* is an advanced asana and requires the spine to be very flexible. If you've had a spinal injury or abdominal surgery, then avoid this asana until you are completely healed. Even after healing, practise with caution. Don't perform this pose when you are menstruating.

19

hanumanasana

(lord hanuman's pose)

Yoga is not only a form of movement. It is a practice that has an emotional, physical and psychological impact on the practitioner. How we work through progressively difficult asanas on the mat reflects how we navigate through challenges in life. Yoga practice encourages students to rethink old patterns and beliefs so that they can move forward in life with courage and strength. The *hanumanasana* encourages yogis not only to stretch beyond their existing limits, but also to overcome fears.

LEAP OF FAITH

When Hanuman decided to rescue Sita, he surveyed Lanka. It lay across the vast expanse of the ocean. He considered crossing it with a single leap, but was plagued with self-doubt. He had jumped large distances before, but a distance of this magnitude . . . Taking a deep breath, he took a leap of faith.

Little did he know that his faith would be tested over and over again on his journey.

As Hanuman flew, it seemed to him that the length he had to cross was endless. Suddenly, he noticed the Mainak Parvat in the middle of the ocean. He was tempted to take a break and rest. Everyone had heard stories of the Mainak Parvat—fragrant flowers, fresh air, delicious fruits. All these enticed him, and a rest seemed like a good idea. But when Hanuman looked ahead at Lanka and saw the remaining distance, he flew on with renewed energy. He remembered he was doing this for Lord Rama, who was like an elder brother or a father to him. Hanuman chose to focus on his goal over the comforts of Mount Mainak.

A little while later, Hanuman was accosted by Surasa, the evil mother of snakes. Her eyes were large and yellow and she had sharp fangs. She was terrifying. She was also the size of a mountain and blocked his way.

'It looks as though the gods have sent you to me as food,' Surasa said to Hanuman. 'I must do as the gods will it, and eat you.' And she swooped down to take a bite of him.

Hanuman jumped back and said, 'Dear Surasa, right now I am on an important mission. I must rescue Sita, who has been captured by the evil Ravana and is being held captive in Lanka. I have been entrusted with this task by Lord Rama, who is like a father to me. I can't disobey my father's command. Please allow me to pass and complete my task.'

'Fortunately, a boon has been granted to me,' replied Surasa. 'You can pass on only through my mouth!' Saying this, she opened her deadly jaws and tried to devour Hanuman again.

Hanuman jumped out of the way and tried to reason with her once more. 'Please let me go and complete my task. I promise, once it's done, I will come back and gladly get into your mouth.'

Surasa remained obstinate. Hanuman started feeling restless. And then an idea struck him.

'If you want to eat me, Surasa, you must devour me whole and not in parts. If you agree to do so, I promise I will not jump out of the way,' said Hanuman.

Delighted, Surasa opened her mouth wide to devour him. As she opened her mouth wider and wider, he started to expand too. Finally, when her mouth was stretched to a hundred times its original size, Hanuman quickly reduced himself to the size of a thumb and jumped into her mouth. Before Surasa could realize what had happened, Hanuman had already jumped out of her ear!

'Now please let me pass, Surasa. I have entered your mouth and have honoured the boon that you have been granted.'

Surasa was impressed, much against her will. She was pleased Hanuman had respected the boon she had been given. She blessed him and wished him success in his task.

Hanuman flew on and could soon see his destination. However, the demons were still trying to distract him and prevent him from reaching Lanka.

As the distance to Lanka decreased, Hanuman started feeling heavy and realized he was slowing down. He felt he was being pulled down by a strong force. Suddenly, he remembered what his friend Sugriva had told him.

'O Hanuman!' Sugriva had said. 'I wish you luck in the noble task you have before you. But be warned! On your way to Lanka, you may meet Simhika, a powerful demoness. She grabs people's shadows and then kills them to eat them!'

Hanuman looked down and saw Simhika emerging from the sea to grab his shadow. Hanuman once again thought quickly. He reduced his size and entered Simhika's mouth. Then he grew to his normal size, ripping her apart as he emerged.

Finally, he reached his destination.

SIGNIFICANCE AND SYMBOLISM

Any big task seems daunting in the beginning. The magnitude of a task shouldn't deter us from trying to complete it. Although Hanuman was brave, devoted to Rama and committed to his mission, he still had to fight distractions. The most focused people can get distracted.

Hanuman also had moments of self-doubt. But because he truly believed in his goal and in himself, he was able to overcome the obstacles that stood in his way. Hanuman took a leap of faith, and so should we whenever we decide to work towards a goal.

Hanuman's journey to Lanka symbolizes our journey to our goals. Just like he was tested repeatedly, we are tested many times in life. Every obstacle we encounter should be treated as a challenge. If we keep our heads and wits about us, it is possible to overcome any challenge. With true faith and belief, we can surmount any difficulty life throws our way.

HOW TO

1. Start with your right foot on the floor, with your hands on either side of it. Stretch the left leg back, keeping the toes on the floor.
2. Begin walking your right foot forward. Stretch it straight out in front of you.
3. Lift the left knee up, and engaging the quads, stretch the left leg until it is straight.
4. Square your hips.
5. Repeat on the other side.

HELPFUL HINTS

- Place a blanket under the foot to slide it forward easily.
- Use a block under each hand. The added height will ensure a straight spine.
- Use bolsters under your thighs if you are unable to straighten the legs completely.

BENEFITS

- Relaxes the mind and increases energy.
- Helps eliminate lower back pain.
- Great stretch for the lower body.

- Strengthens the core muscles.
- Improves digestion.
- Beneficial for the reproductive organs.
- Relaxes the spine.
- Helps to release stress and tension.

CONTRAINDICATIONS

The hanumanasana is an advanced posture and should only be done with proper technique. Make sure your body is warmed up before you attempt this pose. Don't perform it if you have injured your hamstrings or groin.

20

kakasana

(crow pose)

To experience harmony, it is imperative to co-exist with others who don't share our beliefs. Staying true to our intentions, morals and ethics can sometimes be a challenge. Yoga teaches us how to remain true to our values even when the world around us is changing rapidly. Regular yoga practice teaches us how to look inwards to recognize our true emotions and feelings. It cultivates stronger intuition in practitioners, helping them to increasingly trust and rely on it.

Yoga reconnects us to ourselves. True yoga practice is being able to understand ourselves and becoming more self-aware. It seems far-fetched that a pose named after crows could help us cultivate a sense of awareness. However, as the following story shows, there is a reason crows are able to see beyond the surface, and why it is apt that we have a yoga pose named after them.

A CURSE AND A BOON

Life in the forest was new to Rama, Lakshmana and Sita. They were used to the finest luxuries of palaces and couldn't have conceived of the austere life they would soon be leading. They yearned for many things they had hitherto taken for granted. However, they soon got accustomed to it and even started to enjoy the forest. They worked hard and slept soundly. They lived in harmony with the other creatures in the forest. They ate the fruit from the trees and bathed in the clean, sparkling streams of the forest.

One day, while Rama and Sita were resting, a crow flew at Sita and started to bite her. Sita was frightened and cried out in pain. Hearing her cries, Rama awoke. Sita narrated her ordeal and pointed out the crow that had now flown a little farther away. Livid, Rama strung his bow and took aim. He now got a closer look at the crow and realized that this wasn't any ordinary crow. It was Jayanta, Indra's son, disguised as a crow. Rama realized that Jayanta attacked Sita despite knowing that she had Rama and Lakshmana's protection. That made him even more furious and he decided to kill Jayanta.

Jayanta was besotted with Sita and her pristine beauty. Seeing Rama asleep, he assumed that Sita was unprotected and wanted to take advantage of her. Now, as Ram took aim at him, Jayanta became alarmed. He knew Rama was a renowned marksman. Jayanta started to beg for forgiveness.

'O Lord Rama, please show mercy! I let my base passions get the better of me. I was foolish and I realize my mistake. Do forgive me, my Lord.'

Although Rama was still seething with anger, he realized Jayanta was being honest.

'Jayanta, I can see that you are sorry. However, what you did was wrong and you must be punished for it. I have decided not to kill you, but I will have to curse you.'

Jayanta understood Rama's dilemma and resigned himself to his fate.

'Jayanta, your error was that you wanted to create mischief and hurt another person in the process. You saw Sita and decided to make her your target. You could not have done this had it not been for your sense of sight. So I will make it difficult for you to see, so that you may evaluate everything you see carefully. From now on, you will be able to use only one of your eyes at a time.'

Jayant was crestfallen. Rama continued.

'But, because external objects won't be clouding your vision, you will also be able to see those things which are invisible to two-eyed creatures, such as long departed ancestors and unsatisfied souls. Let me give you a boon too: when someone feeds you, it will be akin to feeding and taking care of their ancestors.'

And so it came to be that crows are both revered and reviled in India even today.

SIGNIFICANCE AND SYMBOLISM

By reducing his vision in one eye, Rama was encouraging Jayanta to see and not just look. Jayanta got into trouble because he failed to truly see what he was doing.

When we practise yoga, our intuition and perception are purified. We are able to observe and analyse more clearly. We learn to respond, rather than react, to situations.

Balancing asanas help us cultivate this 'third eye'. When you practice a balancing asana, you are coordinating your strength and flexibility. Balance is initially hard to find, and that makes the asana appear daunting, even impossible.

The crow pose is intimidating for many practitioners. Keeping the gaze fixed necessitates that we perform the pose without physically looking at the rest of our limbs. The gaze must be steady and straight, else balance is impossible. Much like the curse that Rama inflicted upon Jayanta, our gaze in the *kakasana* can be on only one thing—almost as though we had the crow's one-eyed vision. However, because of the mind-body connection that we cultivate in yoga, we can 'see' the rest of our limbs. This connection is key to performing any asana correctly.

HOW TO

1. Squat on the floor, keeping your feet wide apart.
2. Bring your hands into a namaskar and push your elbows out against the inner knees to widen your stance.
3. Place your hands on the floor in front of your feet, leaving about five inches between your toes and your wrists.
4. Once your hands are firmly on the floor, lift your buttocks as high as you can, and at the same time, lower your face to the floor.
5. Lean forward into your arms, securing each knee close to the armpit.
6. Lift the feet one by one.
7. Engage your arms and try to straighten the elbows.

HELPFUL HINTS

- Place a bolster or a cushion in front of you so that if you fall forward, you don't hit your face on the floor.
- Place your feet up on blocks to give you added height. This will give you the feeling of a lift and also reduce the distance you have to rise from the floor.

BENEFITS

- Strengthens the arms and the wrists.
- Tones the abdomen.
- Massages the abdominal organs.
- Inculcates a sense of balance.
- Calms and focuses the mind.

CONTRAINDICATIONS

The novice would assume that the kakasana is purely about arm strength. However, your ability to balance depends on a combination of shoulder mobility, hip and knee flexibility and core strength. Don't perform this asana if you've injured your arms, wrists or shoulders.

21

kapotasana

(pigeon pose)

The origin of some asanas is deceptive. It is popularly believed that the *kapotasana* is named after the pigeon, as *kapota* is the Sanskrit word for pigeon. The posture itself resembles a seated pigeon! However, as we can tell from the story below, kapotasana has a deeper meaning and link to mythology.

THE MOST ACCOMPLISHED ONE

Kapota is one of the greatest yogis in history. He was so accomplished that he acquired all the siddhis that are bestowed upon yogis when they attain the highest degree of proficiency in the yogic arts. The practice of yoga had made him the most powerful, agile and strong being in the universe. He had great wisdom and intuition. People came to him seeking advice. His clarity of thought could simplify the most complex problems. It was said that he was so enlightened, his soul dwelt several feet higher than his earthly body. When he walked, it seemed as though he was gliding over the ground, his feet never touching the floor.

A yogi appears beautiful to one and all, and Kapota was one of the most attractive beings on earth. He had everything he desired. Moreover, he was dedicated to the pursuit of knowledge and studied the Vedas, shastras and yoga diligently. He was always busy and never distracted.

However, one day, his attention was caught by an apsara, a celestial nymph. Kapota was hypnotized. He couldn't stop thinking about her and wanted to know who she was. He discovered her name was Chitrangadha, and she was the most beautiful and enchanting apsara in the world. Not only that, she was also one of the most accomplished warriors on earth. Her mother was Urvashi, another apsara famed for her beauty. Kapota was mesmerized and wanted to make Chitrangadha his wife. However, he was unsure of himself. An apsara had no dearth of suitors. After much hesitation and great thought, he proposed to her. To his great joy, Chitrangadha accepted.

A celestial nymph and the most attractive being on earth made for a most winsome pair.

SIGNIFICANCE AND SYMBOLISM

In the *Patanjali Yoga Sutras*, much has been written about the siddhis acquired by the yogi after prolonged tapas. Kapota was an example of a being who had attained all the siddhis and reaped the benefits.

In the 'Vibhuti Pada', which is the third chapter of the *Patanjali Yoga Sutras*, Patanjali lists the powers that can be acquired by following the yogic path. He calls these the *vibhuti*s or properties of the yogi. These are:

1. He begins to know the past and future.
2. He understands the language of all people, birds and animals.
3. He knows his past and future lives.
4. He reads the minds of others.

5.   If necessary, he can define even the precise details of what is in the minds of others.

6.   He becomes invisible at will.

7.   He can arrest the senses: hearing, touch, sight, taste and smell.

8.   He knows the exact time of his death by intuition or through omens.

9.   He is friendly and compassionate to all.

10. He becomes strong as an elephant and his movements are as graceful as a peacock.

11. He clearly sees objects near and far, gross and fine, and concealed.

12. He knows the working of the solar system.

13. He knows the functions of the lunar system and through that, the position of the galaxies.

14. He reads the movements of stars from the pole star and predicts world events.

15. He knows his body and its orderly functions.

16. He conquers hunger and thirst.

17. He makes his body and mind immobile like a tortoise.

18. He has visions of perfected beings, teachers and masters.

19. He has the power to perceive anything and everything.

20. He becomes aware of the properties of consciousness.

21. By knowing the properties of consciousness, he uses consciousness to light the lamp of the soul.

22. Divine faculties which are beyond the range of ordinary senses come to him because of his enlightened soul.

23. He leaves his body consciously and enters others' bodies at will.

24. He walks over water, swamps and thorns.

25. He creates fire at will.

26. He hears distant sounds.

27. He levitates.

28. He frees himself from afflictions at will and often lives without a body.

29. He controls nature's constituents, qualities and purposes.

30. He becomes lord of the elements and their counterparts.

31. He possesses an excellent body with grace, strength, perfect complexion and lustre.
32. He has perfect control over his senses and mind, and their contact with the lower self or the 'I' consciousness.
33. He transforms body, senses, mind, intelligence and consciousness to utmost sharpness and speed in tune with his very soul.
34. He gains dominion over all creation and all knowledge.

The purpose of yoga is to connect us to our innermost selves. Kapota dedicated his life to the practice of yoga and attained enlightenment. Because of this, he was respected far and wide and could help others whenever they needed help.

It was his attractiveness and accomplishments that made him universally respected and because of that, Chitrangadha agreed to marry him.

HOW TO

1. Start with your right leg between your hands and the left leg stretched back.
2. Walk your right foot to the left and place the right calf and thigh on the floor.
3. The left knee should face the floor.
4. Placing the fingertips on the floor, straighten your torso.
5. Repeat on the other side.

HELPFUL HINT

⚙ If you are unable to sit comfortably on the floor, use a cushion, blanket or bolster under the front thigh.

BENEFITS

- Increases the flexibility of the hips, legs and spine.
- Tones the abdomen.
- Relieves stress.
- Revitalizes and rejuvenates the entire body.
- Stimulates the reproductive organs.
- Opens up the chest, enabling better breathing.

CONTRAINDICATIONS

The kapotasana is an intense backbend. Therefore, don't perform it if you've had a back injury. Also, because it also taxes your hip joint, don't practice it if you are recovering from a leg, knee or hip injury.

Never force your body to go into advanced asanas. Surrendering and allowing your body to ease into asanas is a better way to practice.

22

matsyasana

(fish pose)

The creation of life was Lord Brahma's responsibility, and preserving this creation was the responsibility of Lord Vishnu. For life to continue, everything must work in tandem. This story is about the time Lord Brahma and Lord Vishnu worked together to save the universe.

THE FISH WHO SAVED THE WORLD

King Manu was a great and benevolent king. He studied the scriptures and the Vedas and performed his duties faithfully. He was an ardent devotee of Vishnu and his greatest desire was to see Lord Vishnu with his own eyes. With this aim in mind, he performed pujas for years on end, wishing to catch a glimpse of Lord Vishnu. He was single-minded and dedicated.

One day, Lord Brahma decided to rest. He needed sleep because he had been hard at work for a long time. Hayagreeva, an asura, had been coveting the Vedas for a long time and was constantly looking for a way to steal them. Hayagreeva saw Brahma doze off and realized this was the best opportunity to steal the Vedas. Hayagreeva quickly grabbed the Vedas and sped away. But he was in a fix when he tried to hide the Vedas. There was no safe place to hide them as the devas would be able to spot him anywhere on earth. So he decided to take the Vedas deep into the ocean and hide them there.

Lord Vishnu was awake as Brahma slept and he saw all that had transpired. He knew that if something wasn't done, the Vedas would be lost to the world forever and future generations wouldn't have access to the wealth of Vedic knowledge. Vishnu as the Preserver had the responsibility of preserving knowledge for the future. He dwelt on this problem as he abstractedly watched Manu do his penance. Then he had an idea . . .

The next morning, Manu finished his prayers and was about to offer water to Surya with his outstretched palms. Suddenly, he heard a tiny voice saying, 'Oh, please do not throw me back into the water. The big fish will eat me up!'

Startled, Manu opened his eyes and looked around. He realized the voice was coming from between his palms. Looking into the water in his hands, he saw a tiny fish. It continued to implore King Manu to save its life. Being the good king he was, Manu put the fish in his *kamandalam* and took it home.

The next day, he heard the tiny voice again and this time it said, 'Oh, please, great king, put me in a bigger vessel. This kamandalam is stifling me and I feel constrained and trapped. I can barely move!'

Amazed and surprised, Manu put the fish into a larger vessel. The next day, he heard the same cry. As before, he produced a larger container and put the fish in it. He was growing increasingly puzzled, and was starting to realize that this was no ordinary fish. This fish was divine.

He joined his palms and asked the fish to reveal its true identity. The fish turned into Lord Vishnu. Manu prostrated himself and thanked him for granting his most heartfelt desire.

'Please tell me what I can do to please you, my Lord,' Manu asked.

Lord Vishnu decided to enlist his help to save the world. A great flood that would end the yuga was imminent. He instructed Manu to build a ship and load it with the seeds of all the plants, the male and female of every species and the sages and their families.

'Vasuki the snake should also be put into that ship,' Lord Vishnu added almost as an afterthought.

Then the great flood came and washed away everything except the inhabitants of Manu's boat.

Meanwhile, Lord Vishnu had turned back into Matsya, and gone in search of Hayagreeva. They spotted each other at the same time and before Hayagreeva could gather his wits, Matsya attacked him. Hayagreeva put up a good fight, but he was no match for Matsya. Finally, the asura was dead and the Vedas were safe.

Matsya then searched for the boat, which was now caught in the storm raging over the earth. Using Vasuki, the snake, he tied the boat to his fins and guided the boat to safety.

When the storm abated, all the beings on the boat continued on to the next yuga with the Vedas intact.

SIGNIFICANCE AND SYMBOLISM

When all life on earth was in danger of perishing in the flood, Lord Vishnu, in the avatar of Matsya, had to make a plan to ensure life was preserved. He also had to decide what was important and what could be eliminated. It was a great cleansing of the earth. Similarly, we should periodically also analyse what is important and what can be discarded.

As yogis and human beings, we must have clear priorities. Sometimes, doing and thinking about too many things clutters our lives and minds.

Every once in a while, we need to let go of emotions, things and even people that are not healthy, rewarding and constructive for us. This helps us move forward with freshness and renewed focus.

Just like the years change, seasons change and day turns into night, we must also cyclically cleanse our minds, bodies and lives to fulfil our dreams and destiny.

HOW TO

1. Sit with your legs extended in front of you.
2. Leaning back, place your elbows on the floor. Raise your hips, place your hands under your buttocks and open the shoulders and the chest.
3. Finally, extend the neck and place the crown of the head on the floor.

HELPFUL HINTS

- Use a bolster or a block under your shoulder blades to open up the chest and expand it even more.
- Use a blanket under the crown of your head to support it if it doesn't reach the floor.

BENEFITS

- Stretches and tones the abdominal muscles and organs.
- Removes back, neck and shoulder pain.
- Increases lung capacity and enables better breathing.
- Strengthens the back muscles.
- Conditions the spine and keeps it healthy.

CONTRAINDICATIONS

This asana is an intense stretch for the shoulder and neck muscles. Don't perform it if you have a back injury, and high or low blood pressure. Also avoid it if you are prone to headaches, migraines or vertigo.

23

natrajasana

(king dancer pose)

The king of dancers, or the supreme dancer, is Shiva, he who dances the cosmic dance.

Shiva was the first yogi, and is also known as Adi Yogi or the Adi Guru. He taught the secrets of yoga to Parvati, his consort, and to several other students. Those students then taught others and so on and so forth it went. All lineages of yoga today can trace their origins to Lord Shiva.

One of the most colourful characters in the Hindu pantheon, he is as interesting as he is confusing. The gods relied on him as the destroyer. In the absence of destruction, there would only be creation, leading to the crowding of the universe. The natural cycle of all living things would come to an end and there would be no balance.

ENSURING CONTINUITY

The dwarf demon Apasmara presented a particularly difficult challenge. He represented ignorance. Since ignorance is necessary for knowledge to exist, Apasmara could not be killed. He roamed free on earth and troubled everyone. The acquisition of knowledge is hard work fraught with difficulties, and the gods realized that if he were allowed to remain free, the darkness of ignorance would triumph over the light of knowledge. In fact, Apasmara deliberately disturbed and even tortured those who prayed to Lord Shiva for enlightenment. The gods felt the situation was getting out of hand and looked to Lord Shiva for a solution.

It was a troublesome dilemma. Ignorance is necessary for the propagation of knowledge. If ignorance didn't exist, knowledge wouldn't have any value. Conversely, if the acquisition of knowledge became easy, everyone would possess it. So the solution was not to merely kill Apasmara. There had to be another way.

Shiva understood the gravity of the situation and thought deeply about the solution. Apasmara (and ignorance) had to be controlled. He was so preoccupied with his thoughts that his body started to spontaneously move to the rhythm of the *tandava*. This was the first time Shiva manifested as Natraj and danced the tandava. He danced in all his glory and suddenly, unintentionally, he trapped Apasmara under his right foot. Shiva stood frozen as he realized what had happened. He could feel Apasmara writhing under his foot. Even a slight move would allow Apasmara to escape and ignorance would roam free again. Shiva decided to stay in this posture for eternity. The posture is known to us as the *natrajasana*.

This solved the problem of the world. Ignorance continued to exist, but it would always be overshadowed and restrained by knowledge.

AN EXPRESSION OF GRIEF

The tandava was Shiva's means of self-expression.

It was a well-known fact that Sati's father Daksha was unhappy with her decision to marry Shiva. He begrudged them their happiness, peace and love for each other.

Never one to let things be, Daksha looked for opportunities to insult and hurt Sati and Shiva.

One day, Daksha decided to have a huge yagna to appease the gods. He decided to invite everyone except Shiva and Sati. This was an affront to Shiva. Daksha knew that Shiva's presence was necessary in any yagna, and to hold a yagna with Shiva conspicuously absent was a public insult to him.

Shiva understood Daksha's intentions. But Sati was reluctant to believe that her father would deliberately insult his own son-in-law. She decided to attend the yagna anyway. When she arrived, she realized Shiva had intentionally not been invited and everyone knew that. She was saddened and horrified by her father's cruel sentiments. Heartbroken, she jumped into the sacrificial fire.

When Shiva found out, he stormed to the yagna in a rage. He was livid and started to dance his fearful tandava. Everyone attending the yagna feared for their lives and looked for an escape route as Natraj kept dancing. As he danced, he tore a dreadlock from his head and threw it on the floor, and from it rose the warrior Virbhadra, who would avenge the wrong done to Sati and Shiva.

Soon, all the guests had run away and the yagna had been demolished. But Shiva continued to dance the tandava with Sati's corpse. He was angry and extremely heartbroken. His tandava almost destroyed the world but, finally, Lord Vishnu intervened. He helped Shiva come to his senses and regain his composure.

His pain would never diminish, but Shiva found strength within him to accept the circumstances.

SIGNIFICANCE AND SYMBOLISM

The natrajasana depicts a yogi's approach to life. The Natraj statue has a ring of fire around it and Shiva dancing inside, unconcerned about danger. He doesn't let the proximity to danger dissuade him from his dance or his asanas.

Yogis must strive to be like Shiva, to be diligent and to practise daily despite the distractions and obstacles in life. Shiva dances with light-hearted abandon knowing that the one truth of life is his dance, that everything else is impermanent. As yogis, we must seek the truth and stick to it. We must try to eschew that which is unnecessary and inconsequential.

We can pursue our dharma by fixing our gaze and attention on a higher point.

Another aspect of Shiva's cosmic dance is the idea of cycles. Birth and death, creation and destruction, the end and the beginning, all go together.

We must understand that if we want something new in our lives, then we must create space for it. To create space, we need to jettison what no longer serves us or our lives.

The natrajasana symbolizes new beginnings out of the destruction of the stale, the stagnant and the useless. It is a reminder that we need to supress ego, laziness and ignorance to realize the Supreme Truth.

HOW TO

1. Start in tadasana (see Chapter 8).
2. Move your body weight to the left leg.
3. Bend the right leg and hold the right ankle with the right hand.
4. Raise the left hand so that the arm is in line with the ear.
5. Keep your gaze focused on a point in front of you. This will help you balance.
6. Slowly, start to bend forward at the hip keeping your torso straight.
7. Hold. Repeat on the other side.

HELPFUL HINT

- Initially, balancing is difficult. Hold on to a chair or the wall for practice.

BENEFITS

- Tones and strengthens the legs.
- Expands the chest and enables better breathing.
- Helps in cultivating and improving balance and concentration.
- Massages the digestive organs.
- Makes the spine more flexible and strong.
- Counteracts the effects of sitting for long periods of time.

CONTRAINDICATIONS

Balancing asanas should be avoided if you suffer from vertigo, nausea or dizziness.

24

sukhasana

(easy pose)

Sukha means happiness or pleasure in Sanskrit. This pose is unique in that it is not named after a sage or an animal. A reference to sukha is made in the *Patanjali Yoga Sutras*, a seminal text on yoga. It says,

'*Sthiram sukham asanam*.'

Asana is perfect firmness of body, steadiness of intelligence and benevolence of spirit. (PYS 11.46)

Loosely translated, this aphorism means, 'That which is steady and comfortable is an asana.' Here, the word *sukham* means comfortable. A posture is an asana only if it is steady and comfortable. In an attempt to practise the more glamorous asanas, yoga practitioners sometimes push themselves into painful contortions. However, as we see below, postures are meant to be calm and relaxing for the practitioner.

WHAT IS AN ASANA?

As narrated earlier, after he was inspired by Lord Shiva's dancing, Adishesha spent many aeons in tapas. He hoped to be granted a boon to come to earth and learn how to dance like Lord Shiva. Finally, Lord Vishnu, impressed and happy with his tapasya, granted him the boon he wanted. He would be born to Gonika, one of the greatest yoginis of all time.

Adishesha manifested on earth as Patanjali.

Gonika was ecstatic to have a child. She was a yogini and would teach her son all the secrets of yoga. In this way, Gonika became Patanjali's first yoga guru.

Patanjali soaked up all he could here on earth. He learnt the secrets of Ayurveda and became an expert physician. He cured many people and was revered as a great healer. He was so intrigued by Sanskrit that he became an authority on Sanskrit grammar! He was a trusted source for all grammar-related doubts. He wrote many treatises in Sanskrit.

At the time, yoga was a way of life for everyone and was widely practised. Patanjali became a yoga practitioner and gained expertise in that as well. As he delved deeper into the subject, he realized that because it had hitherto been an oral tradition, there was no formal documentation about it, which led to much confusion about the subject. Inconsistencies and contradictions abounded.

One day, a student asked him, 'What is yoga?'

Patanjali said, 'The practice of yoga is a means through which we can attain enlightenment. Enlightenment will lead to moksha or nirvana.'

The student then asked, 'But how do we attain enlightenment?'

'After studying the Vedas and meditating upon their meaning,' replied Patanjali.

'What is the correct way to study the Vedas?' inquired another student.

'It requires single-minded devotion,' replied Patanjali. 'You must sit for long hours meditating and studying.'

'But sitting all day is boring!' said another student. 'It also makes my back hurt.'

'Which is why you must stay in good physical health! And the practice of asanas ensure that our physical bodies are well-conditioned so that we can continue our studies without being distracted by pain,' explained Patanjali.

Finally, a student asked, 'What is an asana?'

To that, Patanjali responded, '*Sthiram sukham asanam*. That which is steady and comfortable is an asana. When we practise a posture, we should aim to make it steady and comfortable. And when even the hardest posture becomes comfortable, then we know that we are on the path to enlightenment.'

Another student asked him, 'What's the best asana for meditation?'

Patanjali said, 'The *sukhasana*. It is a comfortable posture that can be held for a long time. It keeps your spine erect and you remain alert for meditation. This pose brings sukha to the practitioner by bringing them closer to enlightenment.'

This exchange made Patanjali realize the need to collate the existing knowledge on yoga. He wanted to codify the subject and make it available widely for everyone to study. These aphorisms would help seekers deepen their understanding of yoga and remove inconsistencies and doubts that they may have. Also, students and teachers would no longer need to rely on memory to pass on the knowledge, which would further remove inconsistencies. This is how the *Patanjali Yoga Sutras* came to be.

SIGNIFICANCE AND SYMBOLISM

The *Patanjali Yoga Sutras* is a collection of 196 aphorisms about the philosophy of yoga and is the most widely studied text on yoga today.

Sutra 2.46 states, '*Sthiram sukham asanam*.' According to this sutra, if you don't have a sense of calmness in a posture, your posture isn't an asana and you aren't practising yoga. Many times, we hold our breath or furrow our brow when in an asana, trying to hold it steady.

Frequently, yoga practitioners focus merely on the external manifestation of the asana. We attempt to force our bodies into postures our bodies may not be prepared for. In the long run, this leads to injury and actually hinders our progress on the path of yoga.

It is also important to note that maintaining 'comfort' does not imply a compromise on alignment. Just like we need to resist the temptation to painfully push and contort our bodies, we need to also resist the temptation to stay within our physical comfort zones.

For progress, the practitioner must strike a balance between the comfort of practised moves and the uncertainty of new asanas. Discipline and correct practice alone will take us to the goal of yoga.

Yoga was a means of helping people sit for long hours in meditation. The different asanas keep the body fit enough to sit with no pain. Pain distracts the meditator and retards their progress towards moksha. Hence, being pain-free and comfortable is an essential part of practising yoga and attaining enlightenment.

HOW TO

1. Sit with your legs stretched out in front of you and your back erect.
2. Fold your right leg under you. Do the same on the left leg, crossing the left leg under the right.
3. Place your palms on the knees and hold.

HELPFUL HINT

◉ If you find it difficult to sit on the floor, sit on a bolster or folded blanket. The added height lengthens the spine and helps keep the back straight.

BENEFITS

◉ Strengthens the back, spine and abdominal muscles.

- ◉ Loosens the hips.
- ◉ Helps to focus and enhances concentration.

CONTRAINDICATIONS

Most people can perform this pose. Practising with props will make this asana more accessible if your lower body is excessively stiff.

ushtrasana
(page 129)

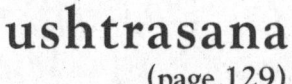

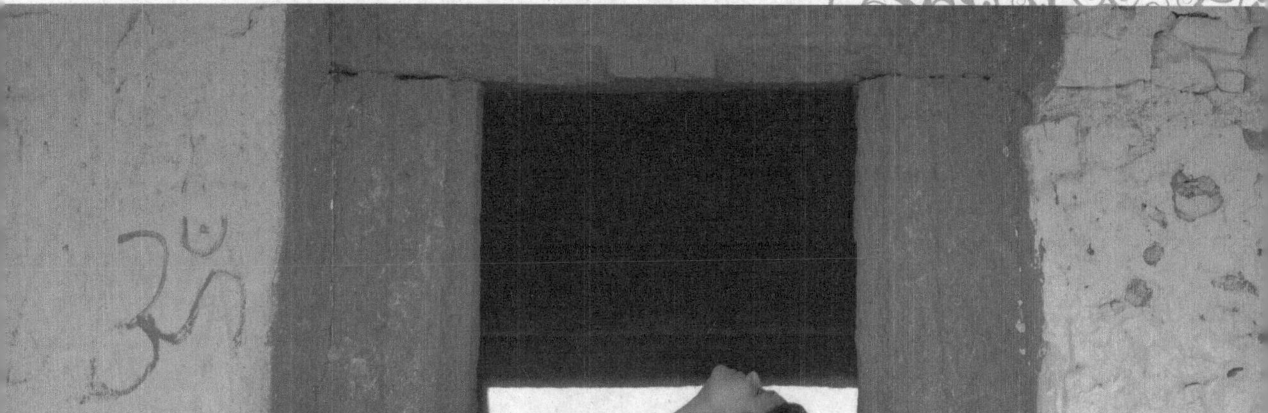

When we understand ourselves, we know what we need. Once we know what we need, we can work towards achieving it.

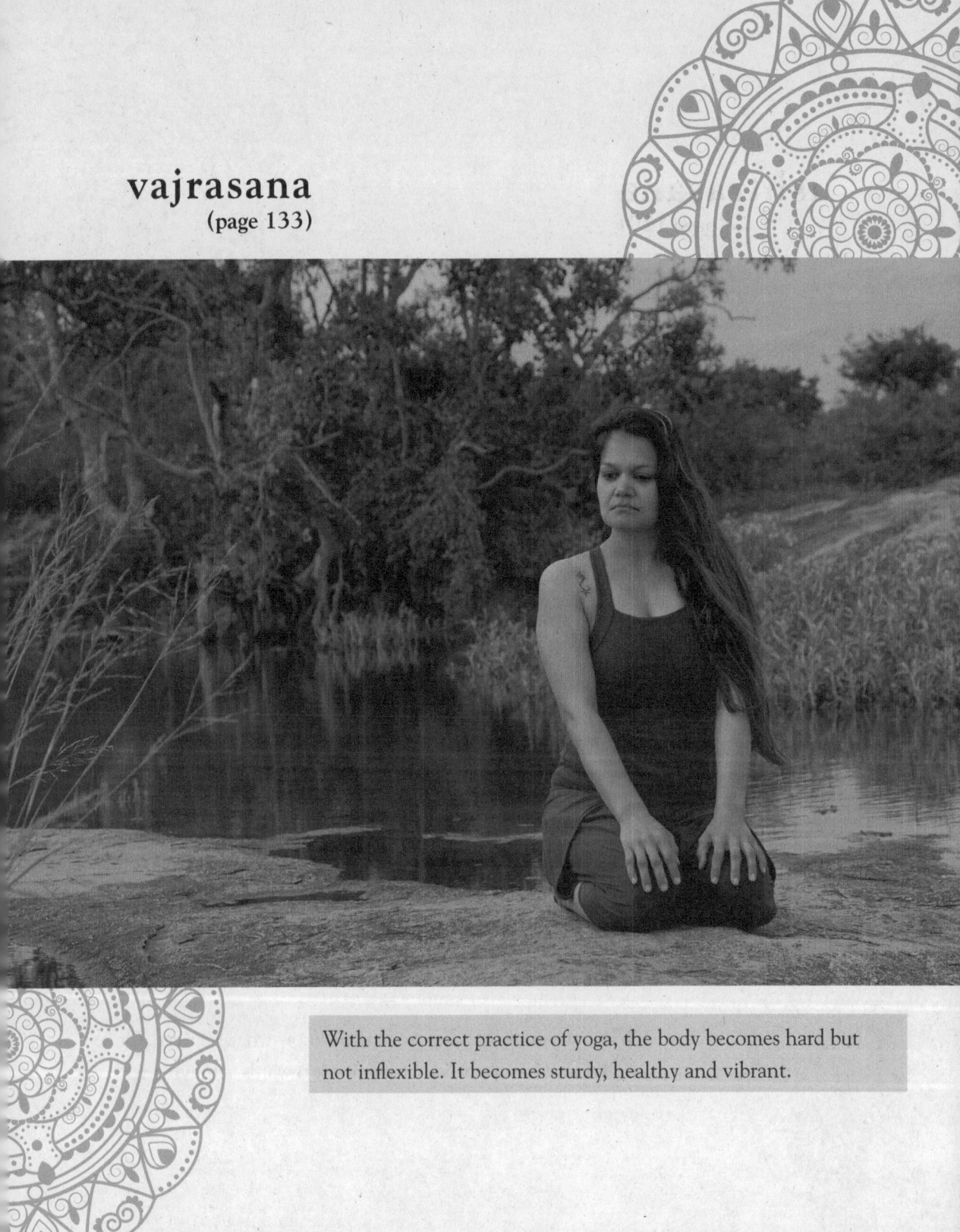

vajrasana
(page 133)

With the correct practice of yoga, the body becomes hard but not inflexible. It becomes sturdy, healthy and vibrant.

vashishthasana
(page 139)

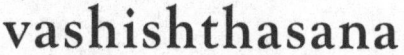

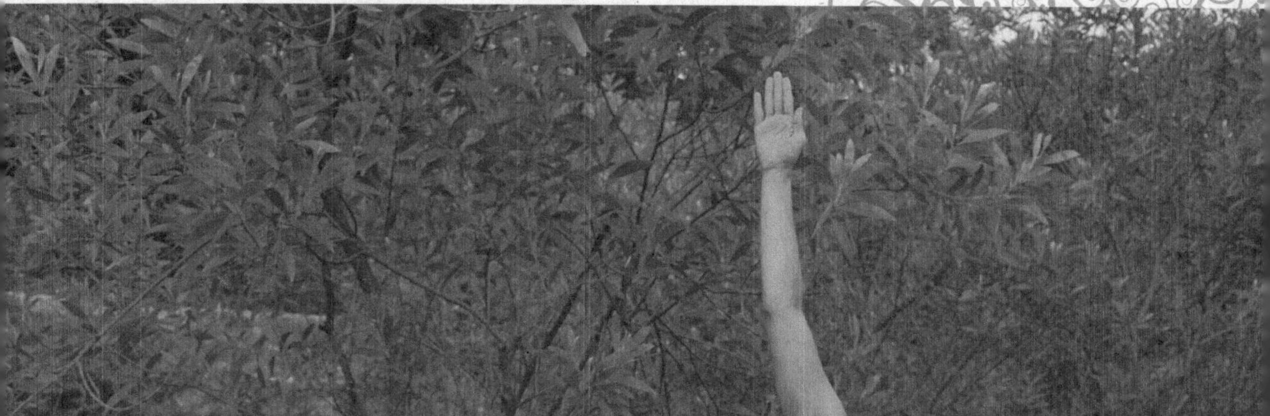

Just like Vashishtha was able to accept the pain in the world and live despite it, we must focus and balance in the asana despite the distractions of our personal lives.

vishwamitrasana
(page 144)

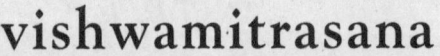

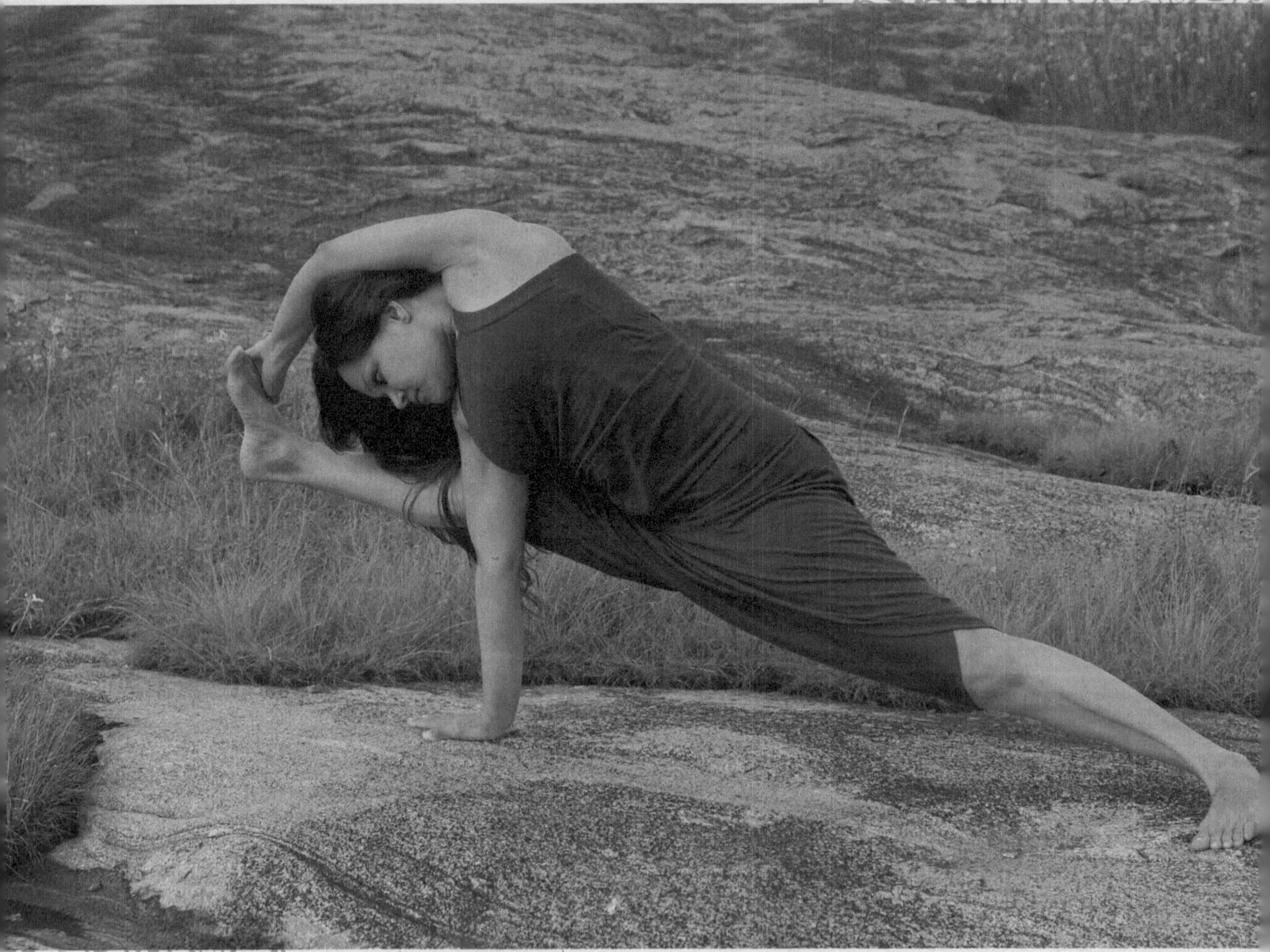

On the yogic path, it is more important to focus on the nuances and the small steps that we can take on a daily basis, instead of aiming for nirvana in one shot.

virbhadrasana I
(page 149)

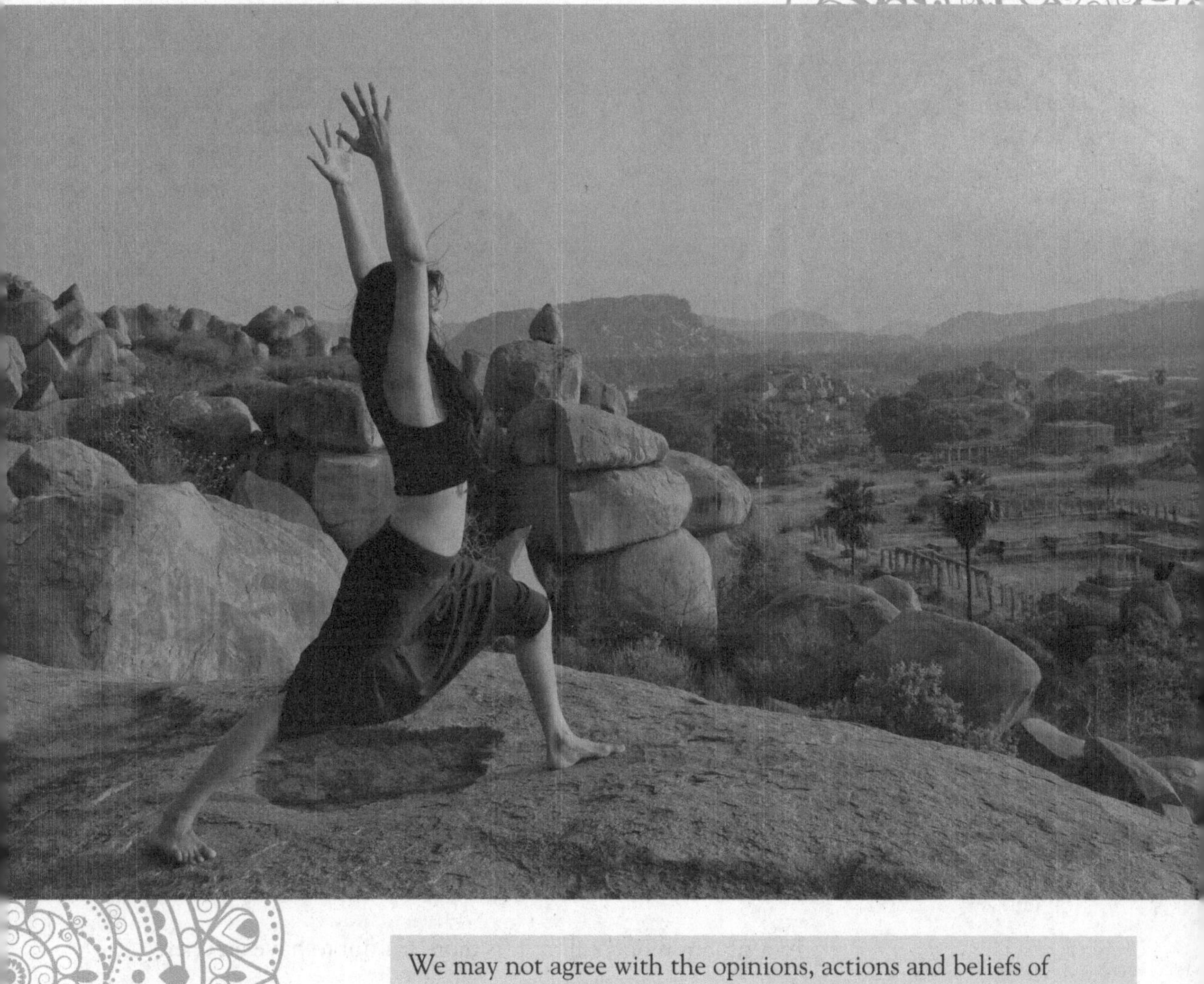

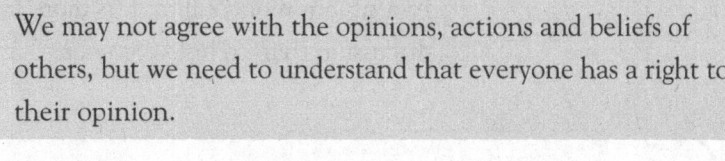

We may not agree with the opinions, actions and beliefs of others, but we need to understand that everyone has a right to their opinion.

virbhadrasana II
(page 149)

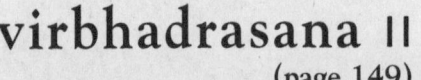

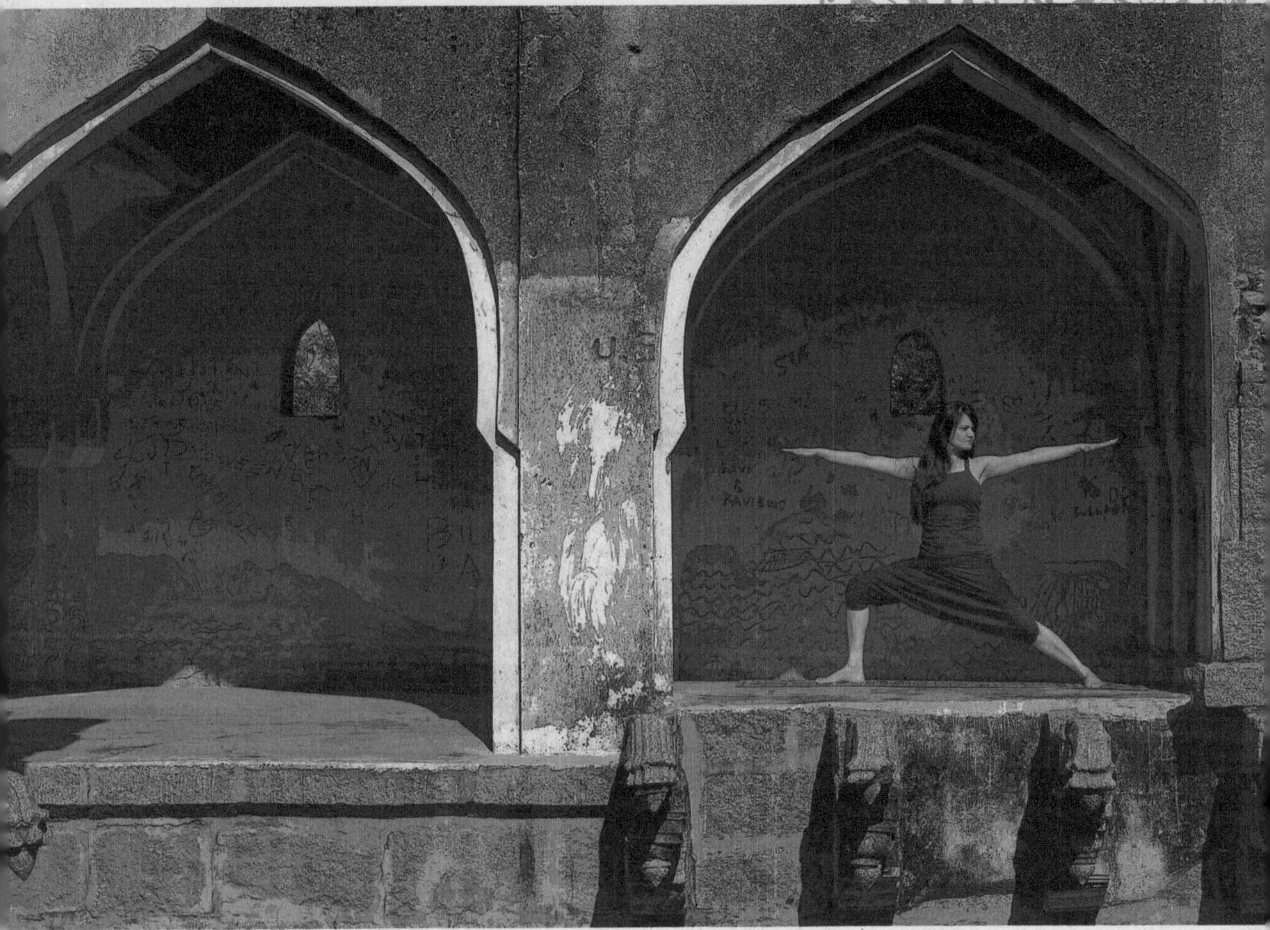

In a situation of conflict, it is more fruitful to have an open discussion than to hold a grudge.

virbhadrasana III
(page 149)

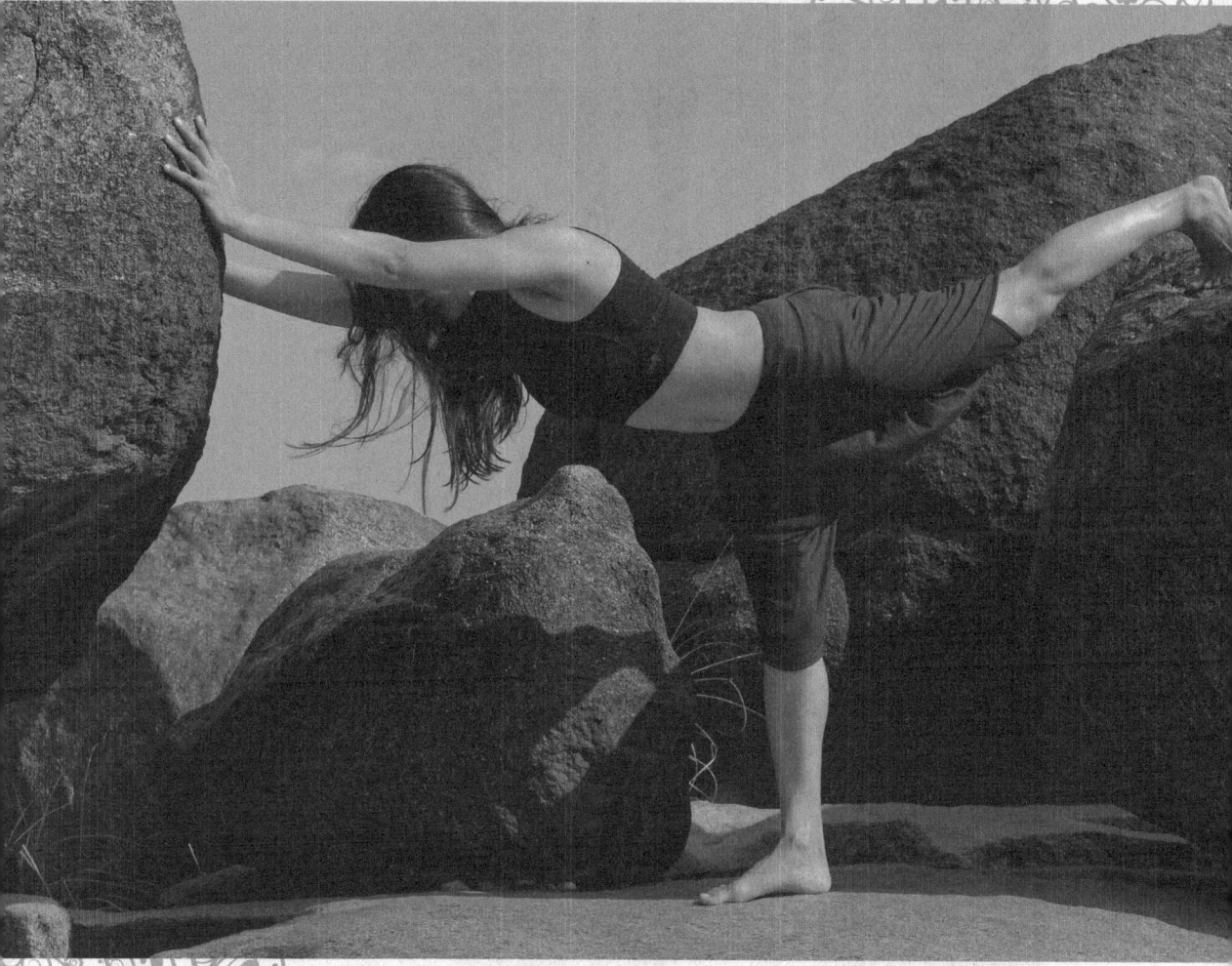

Carrying a grudge is futile and it harms only its keeper.

vrkshasana
(page 154)

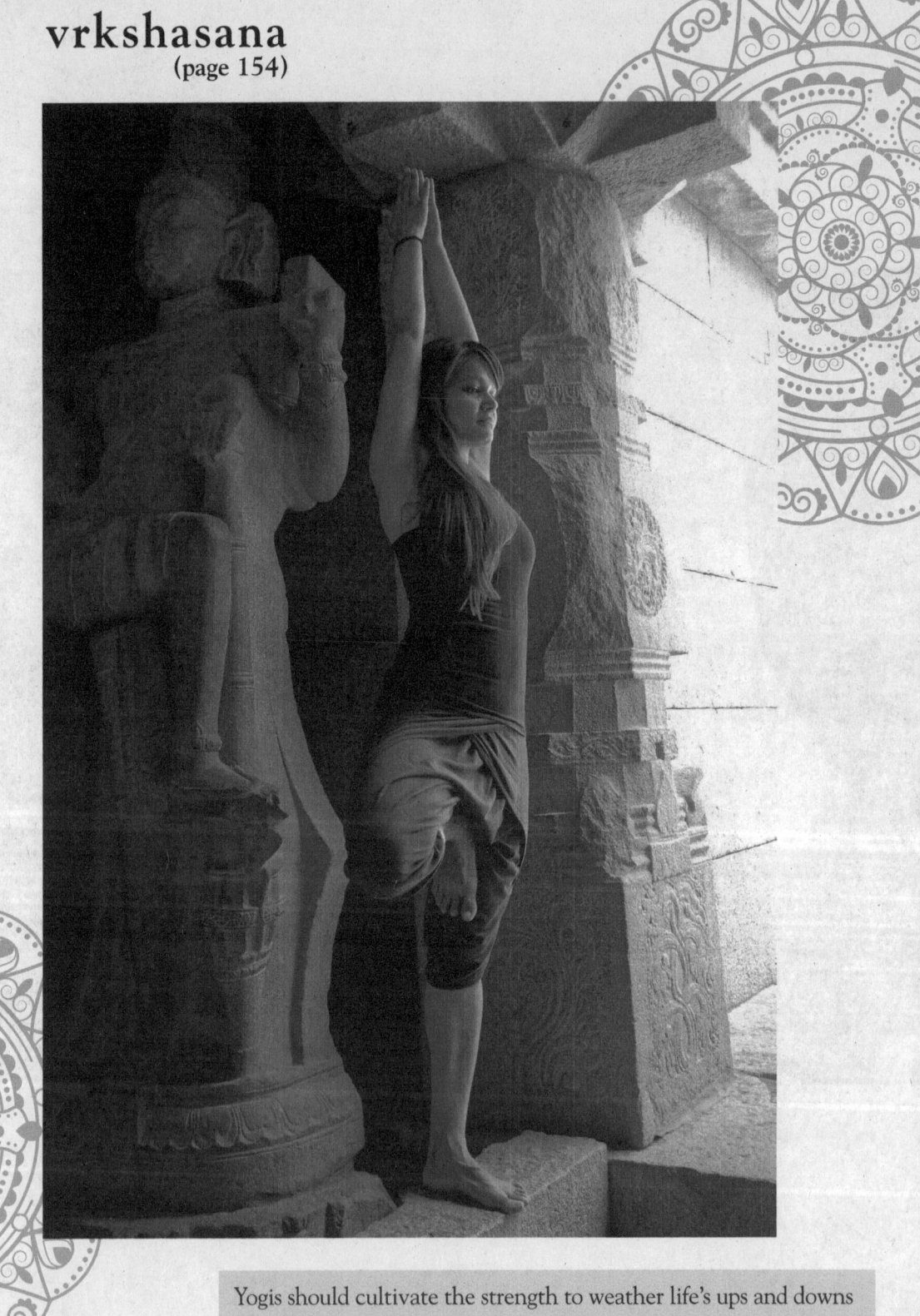

Yogis should cultivate the strength to weather life's ups and downs with ease, without losing their mental and emotional balance.

25

ushtrasana

(camel pose)

The practice of yoga cultivates intuition by encouraging the yogi to repeatedly look inwards and develop a deeper connection to the self. If we want to understand the world, we must first understand ourselves. Asanas work on an intuitive level. Along with the physical impact, certain asanas subtly impact the psychology of the practitioner too. One such asana is the *ustrasana*. *Ushtra* means camel in Sanskrit, and this pose resembles the hump on the camel's back.

THE GREATEST HERO OF THEM ALL

One day, Shiva and Parvati were relaxing in their home. They were talking as they watched their children playing. Parvati was absent-mindedly shaping and reshaping a piece of clay. It was as though her fingers were moulding the clay with a mind of their own.

When she cast a glance at what she had shaped, she realized it vaguely resembled an animal. She started to mould it a bit more. She gave it a long neck and large eyes. She gave it a tail and long legs. The figure had five legs. But Parvati thought it was strangely beautiful with the five legs. The more she gazed at it, the more she desired for it to be a living animal.

'O Shiva, look at the beautiful animal I have shaped from clay with my own hands. I feel like I have created another child. Pity that my creation isn't a living, breathing entity like my other children. Isn't there something you can do?' Parvati implored Shiva.

Shiva replied, 'Parvati, your creation is undoubtedly beautiful and unique. But I think that it will have problems walking with five legs. Look at all the creatures around you. None of them has five legs, and for good reason. It is almost impossible to walk on an uneven number of legs. All creatures walk on either two or four legs.'

'Please breathe life into it. I'm sure it will be able to walk,' Parvati insisted. 'This creature will be a beast of burden. Its five legs will give it a gentle swaying gait and it will carry us from place to place. It will also be used to carry things, even food and water.'

Shiva still had doubts, but decided to give in and indulge his wife. The animal was beautiful, just as they had thought. It was strong, graceful and had beautiful eyes. But it was unable to move! It shuffled forward and backward, and side to side, but never moved anywhere. Shiva realized that it would be cruel to let this animal live. It would have limited chances of survival. It wouldn't be able to run from danger or forage for food.

'Parvati, I feel we must spend a little more time on your creation to ensure that it is self-sufficient,' Shiva said, to which Parvati agreed. She felt that if her creation couldn't help itself, it wouldn't be able to help others. Both Shiva and Parvati put their heads together to see what they could do to help the creature they had created.

After much thought, Shiva said, 'There is enough space in its body to accommodate the extra leg. Let's push the extra leg up, into the body.' Parvati felt that as long as it did not cause any pain to the animal, it was a good solution.

They didn't realize that although its body was large, the internal organs took up most of the space. As a result, the extra leg ended up jutting out of the back of the animal, creating a distinct hump. Both Parvati and Shiva were dumbfounded. They hadn't foreseen this. But to their surprise and delight, this hump allowed the animal to drink a lot of water and store it. It could walk for days without going thirsty. It became the fastest and most convenient means of transportation.

Shiva and Parvati were happy with their creation and proud of its beautiful swaying gait . . . and its four nimble legs!

SIGNIFICANCE AND SYMBOLISM

Taking care of ourselves is the first step towards self-awareness. Camels can survive in the dry, arid heat of the desert only because they have a sixth sense that allows them to find and store nourishment. Like the camel, we should strive to find and store that which nourishes us.

When we understand ourselves, we know what we need. Once we know what we need, we can work towards achieving it. This way, we can take care of ourselves.

Camels store their food and water. They conserve their energy for the long arduous journeys they undertake. Like the camel, we should know what is worth our time and energy. We must remain focused on our goals and not get distracted. Just like a camel fuels up for long journeys, we must assimilate that which we need to achieve our goals. A sense of accomplishment generates feelings of fulfilment and confidence. When we are fulfilled, we are content and live in harmony with the world around us.

HOW TO

1. Start by standing on your knees. Keep your thighs perpendicular to the floor, knees hip width apart and ankles in line with the knees.
2. Place your hands on your waist with the thumbs resting on the tailbone. Start pushing your tailbone forward with your thumbs. As you do so, push your hips forward.
3. Engage your buttocks as you push them forward. Feel the extension on your navel, but do not tighten your abdomen. Keeping the lower body engaged, start to stretch backwards by opening the chest and pushing the sternum up.
4. Place your hands on your ankles and breathe.
5. Look at the ceiling or at the wall in front of you.

HELPFUL HINTS

- Place a bolster on your shins if you are unable to reach your ankles and place your hands on the bolster.
- If you have vertigo or high blood pressure, keep your neck straight and look forward instead of up.

BENEFITS

- Stimulates and massages the thyroid gland.
- Strengthens and stretches the back, shoulders and arms.
- Expands and brings flexibility to the chest so the practitioner's breathing becomes smoother.
- Tones the abdominal muscles.
- Massages the abdominal organs.
- Reduces menstrual cramps.
- Improves posture and problems of curvature of the back.

CONTRAINDICATIONS

The ushtrasana can be a challenge if your back is stiff. If you have a back injury or condition, such as a slipped or herniated disc, don't perform this asana. Backbends should also not be practised if you have a migraine or a headache. Conditions related to blood pressure will be exacerbated by this āsana. Practise it with caution if you have a neck injury.

26

vajrasana

(thunderbolt pose)

Yoga is not just a physical practice, it's a way of life. A yoga practitioner doesn't practise only asanas, but also a code of conduct to attain spiritual enlightenment. As the following stories show, a yogi's emotional and spiritual development are as important as the asana practice. For this reason, ideas of loyalty, fealty, honour, etc. are important on the yogic path.

PAY FOR THE ATTITUDE

Lord Indra was the leader of the devas, the lord of the heavens, and very powerful. He was also the god of the rain and thunderstorms. He commanded a lot of power and because of this got used to getting his way. It was inevitable, then, that before long, his sense of self-importance grew. The powers he possessed went to his head. He forgot the virtue of being humble and started to treat everyone with disregard and carelessness.

Once, during a gathering, Brihaspati walked in. He was Indra's guru. Custom dictated that Indra should stand to show respect to his teacher, but Indra continued to sit. Standing up for your guru is a fundamental rule and to continue to sit was blatantly disrespectful. Everyone noticed this faux pas, but Indra kept drinking and making merry. Brihaspati was stunned and hurt. He had taught Indra all the rules of etiquette and was disappointed that Indra was disregarding his teachings. Stunned, he gazed at Indra for some time, hoping that his former pupil would accord him due respect. Finally, Brihaspati realized that Indra's behaviour was deliberate. Saddened and angry, Brihaspati left.

Lord Indra had hoped his nonchalance wouldn't offend his teacher. His arrogance made him feel that he could get away with such disrespectful behaviour. But when he saw Brihaspati leaving, Lord Indra sensed that perhaps he had gone too far and committed a great folly. Not only was Brihaspati his teacher, he had always helped Indra fight the demons who were constantly trying to usurp his kingdom of heaven. Without his help, Indra would not be able to fight the demons and retain his position as the king of Indralok.

'But I can always ask someone else for help,' thought Lord Indra egotistically. 'I am so important that no one can deny me. Anyone would feel lucky to help me!' Indra continued to be drunk on his conceit.

Finally, the day came when Lord Indra needed help. He was under attack by fearsome asuras and would soon be dead if there was no intervention. Finally, on Lord Brahma's advice, he asked the great Vishwarupa for help. He was hesitant at first because Vishwarupa was half-asura. Lord Brahma assured him that the powerful Vishwarupa was the best person to help. Vishwarupa obliged Indra.

Although Vishwarupa proved himself to be devoted and loyal to Lord Indra, a seed of doubt always unsettled Indra. He was suspicious that Vishwarupa was still faithful to his brethren (the asuras). Years of behaving selfishly with people had left Indra suspicious of everyone. He soon started having petty quarrels with Vishawarupa. One day, the quarrel escalated and Lord Indra was no longer able to control his ugly temper. He killed Vishwarupa.

When Tvashtar (Vishawarupa's father) found out, he was livid. His son's death was untimely and futile and he vowed he would avenge it. He performed a powerful ritual and from the sacrificial fire, the demon Vritra emerged. Vritra's body was indestructible. Tvashtar commanded Vritra to kill Indra. Vritra fought a long and fearsome battle with Indra. Indra was starting to lose the battle and realized he needed help again.

This is when Lord Indra went to Sage Dadichi to ask for a *vajra* (a thunderbolt) to defeat Vritra.

RECLAMATION

Once upon a time, all the devas were driven out of swarga, or heaven, by the asuras. There was a great battle between them and it soon became apparent that the devas were the weaker side. As the battle raged, it become clear that the devas would have to work harder to win this battle and gain entry into swarga again.

The leader of the asuras was Vritra, the king of the serpents. Some say he resembled a serpent, while others claim he was as foreboding as a dragon. He was powerful beyond belief, even more powerful than the most powerful deva. No deva could overpower him. Finally, the devas decided to approach Lord Indra for help.

Indra was a powerful god and very proud of himself. 'How dare they so blatantly disturb the devas?' he thundered. 'I will teach them a lesson they shall never forget. I will face their king, Vritra, in combat, head-on!'

Lord Indra forgot that Vritra had emerged from a very powerful sacrificial fire and therefore, his body was indestructible. Indra repeatedly hurled his most potent blows at Vritra, but Vritra seemed tireless in combat. Try as he might, Lord Indra was unable to defeat him. Vritra was able to parry every blow and continue unscathed. Lord Indra started to get tired. He also started to think that he might need another strategy to win this battle.

Finally, Indra went to Lord Brahma for help. 'O Brahma, you who have created the entire universe! I have been troubled by the asura Vritra for so long. I have employed my best skills to slay him, but he seems indestructible! What can I do, O Lord?'

Lord Brahma, who had been observing the goings-on for some time, said, 'O Indra! You have indeed fought long and hard. Vritra has been given a boon because of which his body is indestructible. It is not your skills that are to blame!'

'But there has to be a way . . .' mulled Lord Indra.

Lord Brahma told him the only weapon that could kill him was a vajra made from Rishi Dadichi's bones. Dadichi was a true yogi and his body was made from the essence of the earth itself.

Although elated that he had finally found a way to defeat Vritra, Lord Indra was unsure of how to ask Rishi Dadichi for his bones. He expressed his hesitation to the devas.

The devas intervened and proceeded to speak to Dadichi on Indra's behalf.

'O Dadichi!' said they. 'We come to you with the hope of a solution to a grave problem. We have been cast out of swarga by the insidious asuras. Lord Indra has been fighting them for us. But the asura Vritra is powerful. We have found out that only a vajra made from your bones will kill Vritra. We have come to ask you for your bones on Lord Indra's behalf. He was too hesitant to do it!'

'O devas!' replied Dadichi eagerly. 'It would be an honour for me if my bones were used to bring relief and joy to people. Peace is the most important thing and I will gladly give whatever is required of me to maintain peace.'

Saying this, he immediately went into samadhi. The gods then used his backbone to create the vajra.

Back on the battlefield, Lord Indra tried to stab Vritra with the vajra, but it wouldn't penetrate him. The fighting raged on.

Eventually, Vritra got tired and started to yawn. Lord Indra took that opportunity to hurl the vajra into his mouth. The vajra was so powerful that it split Vritra into two pieces.

SIGNIFICANCE AND SYMBOLISM

In the *Yoga Sutras*, Patanjali defines the perfect body. Sutra III.47 in the 'Vibhuti Pada' states,

'| | *Rupa lavanya bala* vajra *samhananatvani kayasampat* | |'

Or

'Perfection of the body consists of beauty of form, grace, strength, compactness, and the hardness and brilliance of a diamond.'

With the correct practice of yoga, the body becomes hard but not inflexible. It becomes sturdy, healthy and vibrant. The vajra was so strong and sturdy that it was the only weapon that could kill an indestructible demon. When we perform the *vajrasana*, we must aspire to assimilate these qualities.

Because the vajrasana makes your body hard and sturdy, it is also called the 'diamond pose'.

HOW TO

1. Start with your legs stretched out in front of you.
2. Fold the right leg and sit on the right heel, then fold the left leg and sit on the left heel.
3. Keep the knees and feet together and sit back on your heels.
4. Place your hands on your knees and keep your back straight.

HELPFUL HINTS

- For weak ankles and inflexible metatarsals, place a mat, blanket or a bolster under your feet.
- For inflexible knees, place a bolster, cushion or pillow under your thighs.

BENEFITS

- Helps in digestion and assimilation of food.
- Provides relief to tired legs.
- Alleviates sciatica pain and varicose veins.
- Helps correct flatfoot.

- Helps in correcting the curvature of the back as well as strengthening the spine.
- Eases menstrual pain.

CONTRAINDICATIONS

The vajrasana is hard on the knees and ankles. Perform it with caution if you have knee and ankle injuries.

27

vashishthasana

(side plank/most excellent pose)

Some of the greatest and most enlightened sages were initially as ignorant as the rest of us. Their journeys to spiritual awareness and enlightenment show that the path of yoga is long and arduous, but very rewarding. As demonstrated by the following story, even a sage whose name literally means 'most excellent, best or richest' became enlightened only after going through many eye-opening experiences.

LEARNING FROM PAIN

Lord Brahma was created at the beginning of time. He was then given the task of creating the rest of the universe. Contemplating the enormity of the task that lay ahead of him, he decided he needed help. He would first create beings he could rely on and trust. These beings would then help him create the rest of the universe.

He started by creating four sons. The trials and tribulations that followed have been chronicled in Chapter 13. Suffice it to say that through sheer persistence and hard work Lord Brahma was able to overcome the challenges and create the universe.

Sage Vashishtha was one of the saptarishis who helped Lord Brahma with the creation, and was very wise. Brahma revealed the great secret of mortal life to Vashishtha. He wished for Vashishtha to understand mortal pain and emotions. The understanding of pain would give him empathy and wisdom.

'Vashishtha, I will send you to earth in a diseased body,' said Brahma. 'Only then will you understand what pain is and consequently, be able to transcend it to attain true wisdom.'

Vashishtha readily agreed, but couldn't imagine what he was getting into. Mortal pain was a new sensation for him and he was unsure of what to expect.

The pain got progressively worse and Sage Vashishtha tried to tolerate it as much as he could. But eventually, the pain became unbearable. He wanted a release from the pain but didn't know what to do.

'Maybe, if I do tapas, Lord Brahma will show me a way,' thought a troubled Vashishtha. He started his tapas hoping that Lord Brahma would notice him and he would gain freedom from the excruciating pain of a diseased body.

Brahma finally heard him and decided Vashishtha was ready to learn the great secret of mortal life.

'The secret to enduring the cycle of birth and death is your relationship to pain,' Lord Brahma told Sage Vashishtha. 'The more you fight it, the more it will plague you. Accepting the pain and living with it will help you tolerate it. Then you will learn from it, transcend it and attain enlightenment.'

A WORD TO THE WISE

Prince Rama was destined to become the ruler of his kingdom of Ayodhya. But his real challenge was to become a great king. To be wise, to rule justly and to maintain peace and harmony in the kingdom is no trivial feat.

As was the custom, his training started from childhood. He was schooled in the various martial arts, the art of war, ethics, morality, numbers, etc. However, to be a good king, you must be a good person also. Spiritual evolution was a necessity for a future ruler. For this purpose, Sage Vashishtha was given the responsibility of Prince Rama's spiritual well-being. Sage Vashishtha was the family priest in Ayodhya and he knew (because of his clairvoyance) that Rama was an incarnation of Vishnu.

Sage Vashishtha knew that spirituality could not be learned by rote. He wanted his pupil to have a solid foundation, and that would require time and patience. Sage Vashishtha and Prince Rama spent their days together, learning spiritual lessons from day-to-day happenings. In this way, Prince Rama was effectively able to assimilate important lessons regarding the ruling of a kingdom.

'O great sage!' said Prince Rama one day. 'Everything you are teaching me is priceless and I wish for it to be available to other seekers of enlightenment. With your permission, can we collate your teachings into a book and make it accessible to others?' Sage Vashishtha agreed.

The learnings that were imparted to Rama were put together in a volume called the *Yoga Vashishtha*. It is amongst the most important books in Vedanta philosophy. This treatise is one of the longest texts, the other being the Mahabharata. Chronologically, it comes before the Ramayana. It is believed that those who read the *Yoga Vashishtha* gain spiritual liberation.

THE MOST EXCELLENT ONE

'Vashishtha' means most excellent, best, and rich or wealthy. Being a sage, and one of the most exalted ones, Sage Vashishtha was disinterested in the pursuit of material wealth. He spent his days teaching his pupils, studying Vedanta, preaching karma, dharma and practising tapas. His ashram thrived, his students were happy and there was a general sense of wellness and bonhomie everywhere. Seeing the number of people who were in the ashram, Lord Indra felt the desire to help Sage Vashishtha with the running of the ashram. He decided to give him Nandini, a cow that could grant any wish. Sage Vashishtha was overjoyed with this gift, as Nandini was able to provide food for the thousands of people who frequented the ashram daily. From then on, he could focus on his tapas and teachings without having to worry about providing for the ashram. The cow Nandini was a divine, wish-fulfilling cow. It was the same cow that years later Vishwamitra would desire to own, and which would lead him to one of the greatest journeys of his life.

SIGNIFICANCE AND SYMBOLISM

Sage Vashishtha's journey from pain to enlightenment teaches us that there is a great deal to learn from pain. The path to enlightenment isn't easy or simple. Lord Brahma wanted Vashishtha to learn that pain and pleasure are a part of life and to break free of that cycle, we must shirk neither and accept both. Only this will bring balance to our otherwise unstable lives.

In the *vashishthasana*, we balance on one arm. The entire body has to participate and the mind should be focused to achieve this balance. This pose helps bring the mind and body together, and sharpens our focus.

Just like Vashishtha was able to accept the pain in the world and live despite it, we must focus on our yoga practice and find balance in our lives despite all the inevitable distractions.

This pose inculcates a sense of power and confidence in the practitioner because it requires strong mental focus and balance.

HOW TO

1.   Start by kneeling on all fours on the floor. Lift your knees off the floor.
2.   Place the right hand under your face.

3. Place the edge of your right foot on the floor and rest the left leg on top of the right leg.
4. Straighten your body into a line and lift your hips rather than allowing them to sink towards the floor. Lift the left hand up, away from the floor.
5. Repeat on the other side.

HELPFUL HINTS

◉ Most practitioners complain about wrist or shoulder pain when performing this asana. If you experience pain, shift your awareness to your core and use your core to lift your body.

BENEFITS

◉ Cultivates core and arm strength.
◉ Strengthens the core.
◉ Helps in improving balance.
◉ Enhances the ability to focus and concentrate.

CONTRAINDICATIONS

The vashishthasana is a combination of strength and balance. The more you practise this pose, the more you can hone the relationship between your strength and balance. But if you have an arm or shoulder injury, allow it to heal before you start practising this asana.

28

vishwamitrasana

(sage vishwamitra's pose)

A metamorphosis happens when existing beliefs are questioned and challenged. Sometimes, it requires serious lessons in love and loss for realization to dawn. As we see with the next story, enlightenment comes only after a severe ordeal.

DEDICATION AND DEVOTION

Vishwamitra was one of the greatest sages in the Hindu pantheon. He was born as Kaushika, a great king and warrior.

King Kaushika loved and cared for his subjects and worked hard to maintain peace and prosperity in his kingdom. In return, he was loved and respected by all.

One day, King Kaushika was on the usual rounds of his kingdom when he came across Sage Vashishtha's hermitage. As was customary, Sage Vashishtha received King

Kaushika with the utmost courtesy and left no stone unturned in welcoming him and his army. King Kaushika was extremely pleased with all the arrangements.

'But how can a simple ascetic have so much wealth?' he wondered to himself as he looked around.

Observing the king deep in thought, one of his soldiers said, 'O great king, the secret to all this prosperity is the cow Nandini.'

'A cow?' King Kaushika was puzzled.

'Yes,' affirmed the soldier. 'Nandini was given to Vashishtha by Lord Indra. She is a wish-fulfilling cow and can grant anything to the owner.'

King Kaushika began to covet the cow and asked Vashishtha to give her to him. Vashishtha, of course, refused. The king was livid with anger. He decided to take the cow by force. He declared war on Vashishtha, knowing that a simple sage didn't have the means to combat a well-trained army.

How wrong he was! With Nandini's help, Vashishtha conjured up an entire army of warriors and defeated King Kaushika. The king was awestruck. He realised that spiritual powers are greater than physical might and decided to dedicate his life to doing penance and tapas to gain spiritual powers. He hoped to be a greater sage than even Vashishtha himself.

After many arduous years, his hard work bore fruit and Vashishtha himself bestowed him with the title of Brahmarishi, or the most esteemed rishi. The years of tapasya and meditation earned him the name 'Vishwamitra' or friend of the world.

DEDICATION AND LOVE

Seeing a king become ambitious about spiritual pursuits made many people wary. Lord Indra, sitting in his heavenly abode, became nervous and sceptical. He was suspicious of Vishwamitra and wondered why he was performing such laborious penance and austerities.

'After all, he has a vast kingdom and power, and does not want for anything,' thought Lord Indra. 'So why is he sacrificing it all to live the simple, frugal life of a sage?'

Lord Indra decided to enlist the help of the beautiful Menaka to find out more.

'O beautiful Menaka!' he said. 'Your beauty is unparalleled. It can distract even the most steadfast yogi in his spiritual pursuits.' He shared his feelings about Vishwamitra with her.

Menaka was aware of her prepossessing beauty and the power it had to hold men enthralled. But she was unwilling to misuse it.

'But Lord Indra,' she protested, 'it is a sin to interrupt anyone in deep meditation. And Vishwamitra has spent so much time doing his tapasya that it would be cruel to distract him and bring an end to it now!'

'If his meditations are so steadfast, then he won't be distracted by you,' reasoned Indra. 'And if he is, then he isn't serious about his meditation anyway! An apsara of your beauty is impossible for anyone to resist, though,' he added slyly.

Menaka realized Lord Indra wanted her to interrupt Vishwamitra's deep meditation to foil his plans to become a great rishi. She became curious about the sage whose meditations were a threat to the mighty Lord Indra. Against her better judgement, she decided to see for herself.

When she arrived at the forest, she saw that it was barren. Using her magical powers, she slowly turned the barren forest into a lush, rich jungle. The scent of the flowers in full bloom was enticing and the lush foliage was alluring. Soon, Menaka had changed the mood of the entire forest. Sensing the subtle shift in the environment, Vishwamitra opened his eyes. Incidentally, as soon as his eyes opened, the wind blew Menaka's garments into disarray and she stood in all her glorious splendour in front of him. Vishwamitra fell helplessly in love with her.

As Menaka gazed into Vishwamitra's deep eyes, she also felt strangely attracted to him. She remembered that she was in the forest only at the behest of Indra and his devious plan. But nothing could dim the pull she felt towards Vishwamitra.

'I feel a deep connection to you, Menaka,' said Vishwamitra. 'I would be honoured if you would agree to be my wife.'

Menaka was deeply in love and said yes. They married soon after and had a daughter.

The couple was in the throes of marital bliss. However, thoughts of her original intentions plagued Menaka. She felt guilty about concealing her original intention from Vishwamitra. One day, she decided to confess to him.

'How could you have kept this from me all these years?' thundered Vishwamitra. 'I have loved and honoured you. I stopped the pursuit of higher spiritual goals to live the life of a householder with you. But you have kept me in the dark all these years and taken advantage of my trust.'

He tried unsuccessfully to control his temper. 'I banish you back to Indra's abode. You shall never see me or our daughter Shakuntala again!'

Menaka was heartbroken and pleaded with him to reconsider his decision, but Vishwamitra was adamant.

'I will go back to my tapasya,' said Vishwamitra. 'I now feel I gave it up for nothing. Thoughts of you will torment me, but I am more determined than ever to succeed in my penance and austerities.'

Menaka was helpless. She had to live the rest of her days separated from her husband and daughter. Such was Vishwamitra's dedication to his spiritual pursuits and his desire to become a sage.

SIGNIFICANCE AND SYMBOLISM

Vishwamitra is an example of the value of hard work and perseverance.

Vishwamitra means 'friend of the world'. The only way a mortal king could become a friend of the world is through sheer dedication and single-minded devotion. Vishwamitra pursued his goal against all odds, even attempted sabotage, to become the most powerful sage in the world. His dedication impressed even Vashishtha, the sage whom he had so dreadfully offended. This myth shows that all obstacles, regardless of their magnitude, can be overcome.

Even after years of practice, the *vishwamitrasana* can feel unusual and foreign to the body and mind. To become 'friends' with the asana of the 'friend of the world', we need patience and insight. When we understand the nuances of the movement, the asana emerges naturally.

On the yogic path, it is more important to focus on the nuances and the small steps that we can take on a daily basis, instead of aiming for nirvana hastily. In a similar vein, if we fall off the bandwagon one day, we should move on instead of dwelling on the failures of that day.

HOW TO

1. Start on the right with *virbhadrasana* II (Chapter 29).
2. Place your right hand on the floor in front of your right foot.
3. Lift the right foot and reach across with your left hand to grab the outer edge of the foot.
4. Slowly extend the right leg, but retain a firm hold on the foot.
5. Repeat on the other side.

HELPFUL HINT

◉ For some practitioners, the hips and the hamstrings don't allow for the deep extension required by the pose. Working with variations of the vishwamitrasana will gradually open up your body to perform the full expression of the asana.

BENEFITS

◉ Vishwamitrasana can be done during your menstrual cycle. It stretches the hips and relaxes the lower back.
◉ Helps in stretching the sides of the torso, waist, the hamstrings and calf muscles.
◉ Strengthens the wrists, arms, knees and the hip joint.
◉ Relieves stiffness of the back.

CONTRAINDICATIONS

Avoid the pose if you have injuries on your legs or arms.

29

virbhadrasana

(warrior pose)

The gods and sages of Hindu mythology are upright, hard-working, devoted to their meditations and focused on their purpose. Stories abound of them intervening to right a wrong, or to help a devotee in distress. However, they haven't always been depicted as perfect. Their rage is also legendary and has often brought pain and sadness to the innocent.

Time and time again, they have punished others because their ego was hurt or because they felt insulted. However, as the following story shows, the gods were vulnerable to the emotions of love and pain, and could go to great lengths for them.

AVENGING TRUE LOVE

The story of *virbhadrasana* involves the goddess Sati. Not too long ago, there was a custom (since outlawed) for a widow to end her life by walking into her husband's funeral pyre. This ritual may have started from the actions of Sati, Lord Shiva's first wife.

Sati married Lord Shiva against her father's wishes. Daksha (Sati's father) wasn't keen on his daughter marrying an ascetic. He had hoped his daughter would marry a prince in a lavish ceremony and help him extend his influence and allies. Sati, instead, chose to marry someone who had no regard for social mores, and who was disinterested in the ways of the material world. Try as he might, Daksha was unable to change Sati's mind, nor was Sati able to convince her father that Shiva was perfect for her.

When Shiva's *baraat* (the marriage procession), reached Sati's palace, Daksha and his queen were horrified to see it consisted of creatures from the netherworld! Lord Shiva himself was smeared with ash and had snakes wrapped around his neck—highly unsuitable for a future son-in-law. Sati saw her parents' expression. Her mother was about to faint with terror.

'Please manifest as an avatar more acceptable to them,' Sati whispered to Lord Shiva. 'I want my parents to remember this day as a happy occasion. I want them to be proud of you.'

At Sati's urging, Lord Shiva revealed himself in all his glory. But only for an instant. This seemed to calm her parents down and they started smiling again. However, Daksha had only appeared pacified, but in reality, he was too proud to forgive Shiva's antics.

One day, Daksha planned an immense yagna to which he invited everyone but Shiva and Sati. Sati believed it was an oversight on Daksha's part and urged Shiva to accompany her to the yagna. Sati loved her father and was determined to go. Shiva remained at home.

When she got to the yagna, she realized it was a farce. There were no rites or rituals being performed, and the spirit of piousness was absent. Everyone sat around passing snide comments about her and her decision to marry an ascetic. To her dismay, Sati realized that Daksha did not come to her defence. She understood now that he was still furious she had married Shiva against his wishes. She watched in disbelief as her father joined the others in ridiculing her.

Sati was shocked, saddened and angry.

'All my life I have respected and loved you, Father,' she said. 'I exist because of you. But your behaviour today makes me ashamed to be a part of you, to have come from you. I have a deep sense of loathing for myself now and I wish to be free of my mortal body.' Before anyone could react, Sati stepped into the sacrificial fire of the yagna.

When Shiva learnt that Sati had ended her life, he was grief-stricken and also angry. So angry, in fact, that he wanted to pull his hair out. And that is exactly what he did. Shiva tore out a dreadlock and flung it to the floor in a frenzy. And from there arose Virbhadra. Shiva looked at the fearsome warrior, pleased, and bade him go to the yagna and destroy it.

The different variations of the virbhadrasana are inspired by the different postures that Virbhadra took when carrying out Shiva's wishes. As he got ready to attack, he lifted his hands to the heavens (virbhadrasana I). When he arrived at the scene, he had both his hands stretched to the sides (virbhadrasana II). Finally, he took the position of virbhadrasana III to decapitate everyone at the yagna. Needless to say, there was unnecessary bloodshed, everyone was traumatized and Shiva's wrath came to be feared by one and all. Finally, Daksha begged for forgiveness and Shiva relented. And lo and behold—Sati came back to life as Parvati!

SIGNIFICANCE AND SYMBOLISM

Daksha was never happy with his daughter's decision to marry a man he didn't approve of. Rather than honestly expressing his feelings to Sati, he hurt her by insulting her husband. His actions weren't driven by concern or love for his daughter, but by a desire to avenge a perceived slight to his ego. Had Daksha been more accepting of Sati's decision, or chosen a more forthright manner to communicate his feelings, the terrible events that followed could have been prevented.

We may not agree with the opinions, actions and beliefs of others, but we need to understand that everyone has a right to their opinion. In a situation of conflict, it is more fruitful to have an open discussion than to hold a grudge. To be hurtful and judgemental will not change anyone's point of view. Carrying a grudge is futile and it harms only its keeper.

VIRBHADRASANA I (WARRIOR I)

HOW TO

1. Stand with your feet about four feet apart, toes facing forward.
2. Raise your arms, extending your torso upwards, and expand your chest.
3. Maintain this extension and turn your right foot out. The heel of the right foot should be in line with the centre of your left foot.
4. Now turn your torso so that you are facing the same direction as your right foot (For better balance, turn your left foot about fifteen degrees inwards). Square the hips and shoulders.
5. Bend the right knee and lower yourself until the right thigh is parallel to the floor.
6. Repeat on the left side.

BENEFITS

- Strengthens and stretches the legs, arms, hips and groin.
- Eases stress out of the body.
- Develops core strength.
- Enables better breathing by expanding the shoulder blades and the chest.
- Gives relief from sciatica pain.
- Fixes misalignment of the feet, ankles and knees.
- Therapeutic for flat foot.
- Improves balance and posture.
- Tones the abdomen.

VIRBHADRASANA II (WARRIOR II)

HOW TO

1. Follow the instructions for virbhadrasana I till step 3.
2. Extend your arms to the sides, drawing your shoulder blades away from each other. Your arms should be parallel to the floor.
3. Now bend your knee and lower yourself until your right thigh is parallel to the floor.
4. The right knee should be in line with the right ankle.
5. Repeat on the other side.

VIRBHADRASANA III (WARRIOR III)

HOW TO

1. Follow the instructions for virbhadrasana I till step 4.
2. Keep your gaze fixed on a point and start to bend your torso forward. At the same time, lift your left leg until it is parallel to the floor.
3. In the final pose, your body should make the letter 'T' with the floor.
4. Repeat on the other side.

CONTRAINDICATIONS

All three variations of the warrior pose require the knees to bend and the groin to be stretched, so don't perform it if you're recovering from leg or hip injuries.

30

vrkshasana

(tree pose)

Trees are special in many cultures. In Hinduism, the banyan and the peepul trees are considered sacred. They are widely worshipped and have given rise to many myths and legends. Many Hindu deities are depicted as having close relationships with trees. Krishna has spoken of the banyan tree as a symbol of the spiritual world because the roots of the tree grow up and the branches grow down. Gautama Buddha attained enlightenment under a bodhi tree. Trees represent everything from birth, growth and death to rebirth.

HOLDING DISCOURSE

Lord Shiva represents the ultimate awareness, understanding and knowledge. Not only did he know the secrets of yoga, but he was also well-versed with the tenets of music, wisdom and the shastras.

As the aeons passed, sages, *tapasvis* and seekers worried that the knowledge Lord Shiva possessed would not be passed on to others. Everyone aspired to seek enlightenment like Lord Shiva. The sages got together and discussed this problem. They decided to ask Lord Shiva to impart his wisdom to them.

'O great Shiva!' they said. 'You are so wise and so knowledgeable. There is no one equal to you. Please teach us how to walk on the path of enlightenment. Please accept us as your students.'

Now it was Lord Shiva's turn to be in a dilemma. To be a guru, a teacher, is not a responsibility to be taken lightly. To impart wisdom gathered through the ages would not be an easy feat. It would need time and energy. It would need dedication and devotion from him and his students.

'Please give me some time to think about this,' he told them.

Finally, he agreed to take up this herculean task.

'To impart wisdom, I will manifest in my avatar of Dakshinamurthy,' Shiva said. 'I will continue my own yogic practices and studies in the solitude of Mount Kailash, but I will also teach all those who are interested.'

Lord Shiva looked for a calm, shaded and comfortable place to conduct his discourses. His eyes fell on a large banyan tree. It had ample shade under it and was large enough to accommodate many disciples at a time.

Lord Shiva sat facing the south and all who were seeking his knowledge sat at his feet. He conducted discourses for many hours under the benevolent banyan. The fresh air and the shade of the big tree ensured that Shiva and his devotees could study without distractions. The banyan tree provided shelter to them for centuries. Years of silently looking on as Shiva imparted his priceless wisdom gave the banyan the wisdom of the ages.

The day Lord Shiva manifested as Dakshinamurthy is celebrated as Guru Poornima. As Dakshinamurthy, he is revered as the ultimate guru.

SURVIVING IN EXILE

Lord Rama, Sita and Lakshmana showed great fortitude as they headed out of Ayodhya, but deep within, they were worried. To live without the comforts of the palaces and the kingdom would be hard. To get used to the austerities would be difficult. They could get used to living in simple and clean surroundings, but how would they procure food and survive the harshness of the elements?

As they walked into the forest that would become their home for the next fourteen years, they realized their fears were unfounded. The forest was lush with trees. The trees kept the forest cool, gave them privacy and made their abode beautiful. And if that wasn't enough, the trees were also full of fruits and flowers that provided them with nourishment. Away from all they had known and loved, they came to rely on the trees to give them a sense of security and home.

SIGNIFICANCE AND SYMBOLISM

A great quality of trees is their ability to balance. They maintain perfect balance through all the seasons, stand upright and selflessly provide shade to all with no bias.

> Yogis should cultivate the strength to weather life's ups and downs with ease, without losing their mental and emotional balance.

We must think about others and how we can have a positive impact on the world through our thoughts and actions.

It is believed that this is one of the oldest known asanas. It has been found on coins dating back to the time of the Buddha. Many believe this asana helps to unearth the kundalini energy. When we practise the *vrkshasana*, we try and assimilate the characteristics of trees, characteristics such as strength, rootedness and constancy. In this asana, our legs represent the roots of the tree, our torso represents the trunk and the arms represent the branches and leaves.

HOW TO

1. Stand in tadasana (see Chapter 8).
2. Shift your weight to your left leg.
3. Place your right foot close to the groin, with your toes pointing down. Make sure the knee points outwards, to give your hips a wide opening.
4. Keep your gaze focused and form a namaskar with your hands above your head.
5. Repeat on the other side.

HELPFUL HINTS

- If you're unable to place your foot close to the groin, place it anywhere on the side of the left leg, making sure the knee still points outwards.
- Your hips should be in line with the rest of your body, and not pushed back or forward.
- Instead of raising your arms above your head, you can do the namaskar in front of your chest or stretch your arms out to the sides.

BENEFITS

- Improves sense of balance and the ability to concentrate.
- Strengthens the legs.
- Opens the hips.

CONTRAINDICATIONS

The vrkshasana is a balancing asana and is a challenge for those who have vertigo.
Regular practice of yoga can help improve this condition. Practice with caution if you
have ankle or knee injuries. If you have blood pressure problems, don't raise the arms
above the head; try the other variations instead.

glossary

Arjuna: one of the five Pandava brothers.

Asuras: divine beings who are always competing with the devas for power. They are different from the rakshasas, who are simply ghosts and not divine.

Brahma–Vishnu–Shiva: the Hindu triumvirate. Brahma is the Preserver, responsible for ensuring that the universe continues. Vishnu is the Creator, responsible for all creation. Shiva is the Destroyer, responsible for destruction needed to maintain a balance in the universe.

Dakshina: The stipend or fee paid to brahmanas.

Devas: divine beings. Distinct from the asuras in their ability to know right from wrong and follow the righteous path.

Dharma: a set of rules and a code of ethical conduct, appropriate customs and behaviour, duty, rights, character, vocation and religion.

Draupadi: daughter of King Drupad and wife to the five sons of King Pandu with his wife Kunti.

Durvasa: son of Sage Atri. He was known for being very short-tempered.

Duryodhan: the eldest Kaurava.

Hanuman: the 'monkey god'. He is known to be brave, devoted, loyal and chaste. He is also known to patronize the martial arts, acrobatics and even meditation. Plays a central role in the Ramayana and is mentioned in other religious texts as well.

Indra: deity that rules over heaven. Wields a thunderbolt (vajra) and rides a white elephant called Airavata.

Kamandalam: oblong water pot that Hindu ascetics and yogis use to store water.

Kauravas: the descendants of King Dhritarashtra with his queen Gandhari. Gandhari was given a boon by Sage Vyasa that she would have one hundred sons as powerful as her husband. These hundred sons and one daughter came to be known as the Kauravas.

Mahabharata: one of the two Hindu epics. It details the Kurukshetra war and the fates of the Kauravas and Pandavas.

Menaka: one of the most beautiful apsaras or celestial nymphs.

Moksha: to attain freedom from the cycle of birth and death. Also known as mukti.

Mount Kailash: also known as Kailash Parvat. Abode of Lord Shiva and his consort, Parvati.

Mount Mandara: in some texts the mountain is also called Mount Meru.

Mukti: see moksha.

Nirvana: same as moksha.

Pandavas: the descendants of King Pandu by his wives Kunti and Madri. The Pandavas who play the most significant role in the Mahabharata are Yudhishthira, Bheema, Arjuna, Nakula and Sahadeva.

Ramayana: one of the two Hindu epics. It is about the rescue of Sita by Prince Rama with the help of Hanuman and his army of monkeys.

Ravana: often considered the 'villain' of the Ramayana, he kidnaps Sita.

Rig Veda: the oldest Veda.

Rishi: a sage or seer.

Samadhi: the final stage in yoga, where you achieve union with the divine.

Samudra Manthan: once, when the devas had lost their power, Vishnu had alerted them to the nectar of immortality found deep in the ocean. Upon imbibing this nectar, the devas would regain their divine power. The devas and asuras decided to work together to churn the ocean to make the nectar rise up out of it.

Shastras: texts that address a specific area of study. Form a part of the earliest known Indian scriptures.

Siddhis: powers believed to be achieved through long, dedicated practice of yoga.

Sita: Rama's wife, considered to be a paragon of wifely virtues.

Sugriva: son of Surya (sun god) and the king of the monkey army.

Swayamvar: the custom of choosing a husband from among an assembly of suitors by a girl (usually from a noble family). The candidates would typically have to compete with others in a challenge, the winner of which would be the girl's groom.

Tandava: divine dance performed by Lord Shiva. The dance is considered to be the source of the cycle of creation, preservation and destruction.

Tapas/Tapasya: process of physical control and purification.

Tapasvi: those who perform tapas.

Vimana: flying chariots or palaces. Ravana owned the famed Pushpaka Vimana or the flowery chariot.

Vedas: texts that form a part of the earliest Indian scriptures.

Vedanta: a spiritual philosophy based on the teaching in the Upanishads.

Yagna: A Vedic tradition where a deity was worshipped, typically with offerings and sacrifices in front of a sacred fire.

Yug/yuga: loosely translated, it is a Sanskrit term to signify an epoch or an era according to the Hindu idea of time.

acknowledgements

Most of this book was written perched on my chair at a little desk in the tiny apartment I rent on the third floor of an old colonial building in Bengaluru. This being my first book, the task was a little bewildering. It would not have been possible had it not been for the support of a few people who went out of their way to help me—Geetanjali Joshi, Devashish Sharma and Keshav Karna. Their help, support and unflinching belief were important for me during the writing of this book. I also have to thank my sister Kakuli Bhatt for giving me a desk tiny enough to fit in my tiny apartment.

Joel and I are also grateful to Vishnu Naryan for graciously allowing us to use his farm to shoot some of the images featured in this book.

We would also like to thank Proyog for the elegant apparel they provided for the photos illustrating this book. Proyog is a yoga wear brand intent on showing to the world India's competence to design and manufacture best-in-class products. It offers a contemporary rendition of traditional dressing styles, with a focus on comfort and performance.

And last, but not least, a very special thanks to Suhail Mathur of The Book Bakers literary agency for making this book happen.

references

What is Yoga?

B.K.S. Iyengar, *Light on the Yoga Sutras of Patanjali* (Thomson Press India Ltd., 1993 pp 3–9)

B.K.S. Iyengar, *Light on Yoga* (Thomson Press India Ltd., 1993 pp 31–52)

Anjaneyasana

B.K.S. Iyengar, *Yoga: The Path to Holistic Health* (DK, 2008)

Alanna Kaivalya and Arjuna van der Kooj, *Myths of the Asanas* (Jaico, 2014)

Zo Newell, 'The Mythology Behind Anjaeyasana (Low Lunge)', https://yogainternational.com/article/view/the-mythology-behind-anjaneyasana-low-lunge

Balasana

'Top 15 Childhood Krishna Stories for Kids', https://parenting.firstcry.com/articles/top-15-childhood-krishna-stories-kids/

'The Story of Eklavya and Dronacharya', https://wisdom.srisriravishankar.org/story-eklavya-devotion/

'Home Page of Eklavya', http://www.mantraonnet.com/eklavya.html

Ramesh Menon, *The Mahabharata: A Modern Rendering, Volume 1* (iUniverse Inc., 2006)

Trikonasana

'Mahishasura', https://en.wikipedia.org/wiki/Mahishasura

Shivpreet Singh, 'Story of Brahma and the Pillar of Light (from the Shiva Purana) (2011), http://shivsangels.blogspot.com/2011/06/story-of-brahma-and-pillar-of-light.html

Ardha Chandrasana

Divya Chauhan, '9 Fascinating Stories about the Legend of Shiva You Need to Read Today', ScoopWhoop, https://www.scoopwhoop.com/Interesting-Legends-About-Lord-Shiva/#.d5zpw6tqy

Vivek Kumar, 'Why Shiva Has a Moon on His Head', Speakingtree.
in, https://www.speakingtree.in/allslides/why-shiva-has-moon-on-his-
head/302419

Swarajya, 'Samudra Manthan', http://creative.sulekha.com/samudra-
manthan-the-story-read-in-wikipedia_602459_blog

'Ganesha and the Moon', http://hindumythologyforgennext.blogspot.
com/2012/01/ganesha-and-moon.html

Ardha Matsyendrasana

'Matsyendra', https://en.wikipedia.org/wiki/Matsyendra

'Matsyendranath, the Fish', https://jivamuktiyoga.com/fotm/
matsyendranath-the-fish/

Sadhguru, 'Yoga Originated from Shiva', Timesofindia.com (2009),
https://timesofindia.indiatimes.com/Yoga-originated-from-Shiva/
articleshow/4170824.cms

George Weston Briggs, *Gorakhnath and the Kanphata Yogis* (Oxford
University Press, 1938)

Kurmasana

'Durvasa', https://en.wikipedia.org/wiki/Durvasa#Role_In_The_
Churning_Of_The_Ocean

'Samudra Manthan and Science', Speakingtree.in, https://www.speakingtree.in/allslides/samudra-manthan-and-science-302127/118024

'Symbolism of Ksheera Sagara Manthan', https://www.hinduwebsite.com/churning.asp

'Kashyapa', https://en.wikipedia.org/wiki/Kashyapa

https://sagarworld.com/blog/hinduism/puranas-hindu-mythology/ramayan-ramanand-sagar/ramayan-characters/brahma-creator-universe/

Tadasana

'Himavat', https://en.wikipedia.org/wiki/Himavat

'Himavat', *Encyclopedia of Hinduism*, http://hinduism.enacademic.com/325/Himavat

'The Relationship between Mother Kali and Lord Shiva', http://www.writespirit.net/spirituality/the-cosmic-gods/the-relationship-between-mother-kali-and-lord-shiva/

Garudasana

'Garuda', http://deity-of-the-week.blogspot.com/2011/11/garuda.html

'The Birth of Garuda', *Indian Mythology*, http://www.apamnapat.com/articles/StoriesFromMahabharata400.html

'Jatayu', https://en.wikipedia.org/wiki/Jatayu

'Jatayu's Good Fortune', TheHindu.com (2011), https://www.thehindu.com/features/friday-review/religion/jatayus-good-fortune/article2726587.ece

Gomukhasana

'The Story of Nandi', https://www.rudraksha-ratna.com/articles/story-of-nandi

'Nandi, the Vehicle of Lord Shiva', http://hindumythologyforgennext.blogspot.com/2011/12/nandi-vehicle-of-lord-shiva.html

'Vasishta and Vishwamitra', http://www.apamnapat.com/articles/StoriesFromMahabharata660.html

'Kamadhenu', https://en.wikipedia.org/wiki/Kamadhenu

B.K.S. Iyengar, *The Illustrated Light on Yoga* (HarperCollins, 1997)

Ashtavakrasana

S.A. Krishnan, *Ashtavakra: Stories from Hindu Puranas* (Kindle Ed., 2018)

'Raja Janak and Muni Ashtavakra', http://theinnerworld.in/spirituality/from-the-puranas/raja-janak-muni-ashtavakra/

Virasana

'Hanuman Brings Sanjeevani Buti', http://shree-hanuman.blogspot.com/2013/07/hanuman-brings-sanjeevani-buti.html

Marichyasana

'Brahma: The Creator of the Universe in Hindu Mythology', https://www.speakingtree.in/allslides/brahma-the-creator-of-the-universe-in-hindu-mythology-644248/first-creationsanat-kumar

'Marichi', https://en.wikipedia.org/wiki/Marichi

https://www.yogalaurent.com/mythology-behind-marichyasana-pose-dedicated-sage-marichi/

Padmasana

'Hindu Views on Evolution', https://en.wikipedia.org/wiki/Hindu_views_on_evolution

'Brahma', https://en.wikipedia.org/wiki/Brahma

'Padma Purana', https://en.wikipedia.org/wiki/Padma_Purana

Bhardwajasana

'The Story of Bharadvajasana', *Maitri Yoga*, http://yogamaitricenter.com/the-story-of-bharadvajasana/

Bhujangasana

B.K.S. Iyengar, *Light on the Yoga Sutras of Patanjali* (Thomson Press India Ltd., 1993)

Dhanurasana

'Pinaka (Hinduism)', https://en.wikipedia.org/wiki/Pinaka_(Hinduism)

'Draupadi's Swayamvara', http://www.indianmirror.com/history/mahabharatha/draupadis-swayamvara.html

'The Eye of the Bird', http://hindumythologyforgennext.blogspot.com/2013/03/the-eye-of-bird.html

Halasana

Peter Sterios, 'Heal Thyself Head to Toe: Plow Pose', *Yoga Journal* (2007), https://www.yogajournal.com/practice/halasana

'Samba (Krishna's Son)', https://en.wikipedia.org/wiki/Samba_(Krishna%27s_son)

Ganesh Narasimhan, 'Conducting Samba Marriage and Defeating Kauravas' (2014), http://tostrength.blogspot.com/2010/11/conducting-samba-marriage-and-defeating.html

Hanumanasana

'Surasa, the Mother of Snakes Tests Hanuman', Speakingtree.in (2007), https://www.speakingtree.in/blog/surasa-the-mother-of-snakes-tests-hanuman

'Simhika', https://en.wikipedia.org/wiki/Simhika

'Lord Hanuman and Mainak Parvat' (2015), https://www.onlinetemple.com/blogs/updates/16730104-lord-hanuman-and-mainak-parvat

Kakasana

'Jayanta', https://en.wikipedia.org/wiki/Jayanta

Madhavi Rathod, 'The Crow's Significance in Indian Mythology', Vedichealing.com (2014), https://vedichealing.com/the-crows-significance-in-indian-mythology/

Kapotasana

B.K.S. Iyengar, *Light on the Yoga Sutras of Patanjali*, (Harper Element, 1993, p. 36–37)

Sandra Anderson and Pandit Rajmani Tigunait, 'Kapotasana: Pigeon Pose', Yogainternational.com, https://yogainternational.com/article/view/kapotasana-pigeon-pose

Ann Siebert, 'Story behind the Pose: Kapotasana' (2017), http://www.rockclimbingyogi.com/blog/story-behind-the-pose-kapotasana

Matsyasana

'Lord Vishnu's Matsya Avtaar Story', http://krishnaseva.blogspot.com/2014/06/lord-vishnus-matsya-avtaar-story.html

'Matsya Avatar', http://hindumythologyforgennext.blogspot.com/2011/11/matsya-avatar.html

Natrajasana

Divya Chauhan, '9 Fascinating Stories about the Legend of Shiva You Need to Read Today', ScoopWhoop.com (2016), https://www.scoopwhoop.com/Interesting-Legends-About-Lord-Shiva/#.dvq44hna0\

'Apasmara', https://en.wikipedia.org/wiki/Apasmara

'Shiva Tandav Dance: Why Did Lord Shiva Perform Tandava?', https://www.tentaran.com/shiva-tandav-dance-lord-shiva/

Sukhasana

'The Legend of Sage Patanjali', http://bksiyengar.com/modules/iyoga/legend.htm

Ushtrasana

Pallav Pahuja, 'Camels and Camel Keepers of the Thar Desert' (2017), http://sujanluxury.com/blog/2017/11/17/camels-and-camel-keepers-of-the-thar-desert/

Vajrasana

SB 6.7: 'Indra Offends His Spiritual Master, Bṛhaspati', https://www.vedabase.com/en/sb/6/7/chapter-view

'Indra and Vritra Part 1 of 2', http://hindumythologyforgennext.blogspot.com/2011/12/indra-and-vritra-part-1.html

'Dadhichi', https://en.wikipedia.org/wiki/Dadhichi

Vashishthasana

YJ Editors, 'SidePlank Pose', Yogajournal.com (2007), https://www.yogajournal.com/poses/side-plank-pose

'Yogi Vasishta', https://en.wikipedia.org/wiki/Yoga_Vasistha

Rajeev Singh, 'Rishi Vasista—Who Was Full of Compassion Even towards His Enemies', Detechter.com, https://detechter.com/sage-vasistha-who-was-full-of-compassion-even-towards-his-enemies/

Valmiki, *Yoga Vashishtha*, https://www.slideshare.net/pard57/yv-bkii-ch10-brahma-propounds-the-knowledge-of-liberation-to-vashishtha: Sehgal Pradeep, April 16, 2016.

'Lord Brahma: The God of Creation', https://www.thoughtco.com/lord-brahma-the-god-of-creation-1770300

'Kamadhenu', https://en.wikipedia.org/wiki/Kamadhenu

Vishwamitrasana

'Vishwamitra—The King Who Became a Great Sage', http://www.apamnapat.com/entities/Vishwamitra.html

Arshia Sattar, 'The Ultimate Male Fantasy', TheHindu.com (2017), https://www.thehindu.com/society/history-and-culture/analysing-the-episode-of-apsara-menaka-and-sage-vishwamitra/article19125560.ece

'Vishwamitra and Menaka', http://www.kidsgen.com/fables_and_fairytales/indian_mythology_stories/vishwamitra_and_menaka.htm

Virbhadrasana

'Warrior Poses' (2002), https://jivamuktiyoga.com/fotm/warrior-poses/

Utkarsh Patel, 'Lord Shiva's Wedding Procession' (2011), http://utkarshspeak.blogspot.com/2011/03/lord-shivas-wedding-procession.html

Vrkshasana

'Dakshinamurthy', https://en.wikipedia.org/wiki/Dakshinamurthy

a note on the author

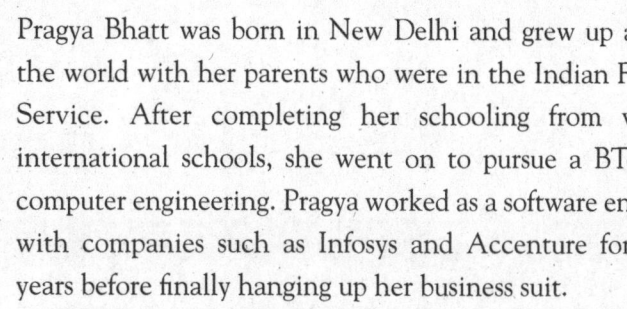

Pragya Bhatt was born in New Delhi and grew up around the world with her parents who were in the Indian Foreign Service. After completing her schooling from various international schools, she went on to pursue a BTech in computer engineering. Pragya worked as a software engineer with companies such as Infosys and Accenture for eight years before finally hanging up her business suit.

After receiving her Yoga Instructors' Certification from SVYASA (Swamy Vivekananda Yoga Anusudhana Samsthana), she continues to deepen her practice under the guidance of noted teachers. She conducts group and private classes, international trainings and retreats. Her teachings are also available online at www.yogawithpragya.com.

Pragya Bhatt lives in Bangalore, India. A quintessential Third Culture Kid, she has a keen interest in art, culture, literature and travel. This is her first book.

a note on the photographer

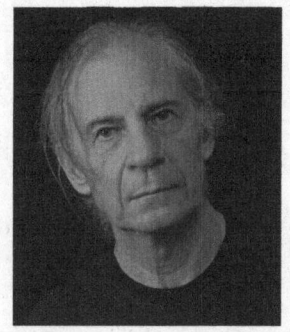

Joel Koechlin was born in France but has spent most of his life in India. Educated in photography at Switzerland's prestigious École Supérieure d'Arts Appliqués—the Advanced School of Applied Arts—he has fostered an unwavering passion for the craft over several decades.

He began his career as a professional photographer in advertising agencies in Paris, France, and has continued as a freelance photographer in India, from Bangalore to the high Himalayas. He has covered a variety of subjects, extending from architectural and corporate photography to adventure and travel articles for magazines. He is a pilot, a motorcycle enthusiast, a mountain lover and a freelance author, prompt to embrace all aspects of life, in a perpetual quest for personal development and progress. His wife is Indian and he has two children.

His work is accessible online at www.lumieres-india.com.